sakara (suh-KAR-uh), Sanskrit, *adj*.: With form. Or giving form to that which does not have form. *n*.: The action of turning thoughts to things and dreams into reality. What I think I create.

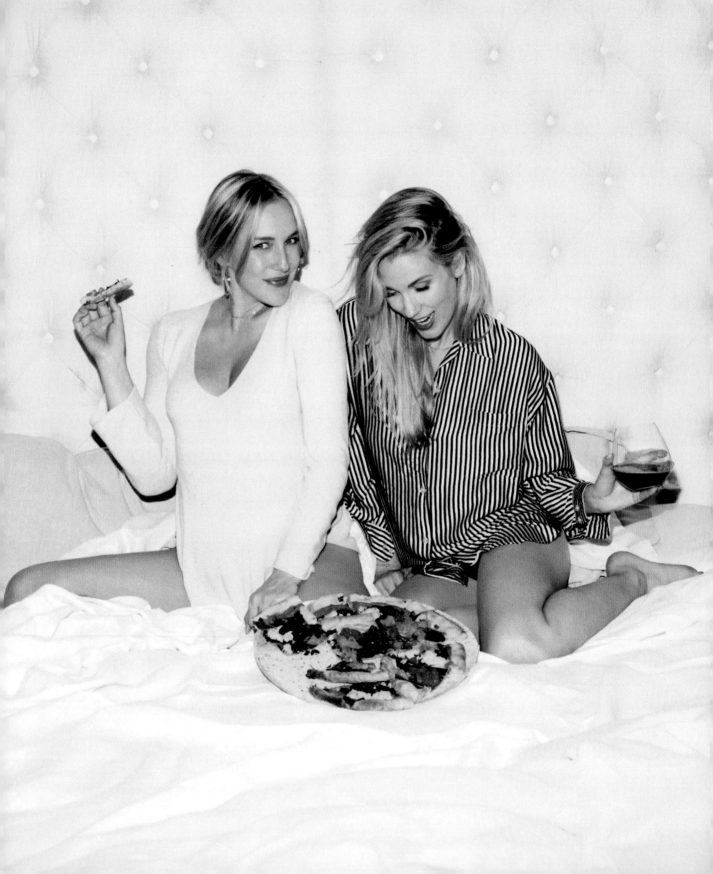

EAT CLEAN PLAY DIRTY

RECIPES FOR A BODY AND LIFE YOU LOVE

DANIELLE DUBOISE + WHITNEY TINGLE
FOUNDERS OF SAKARA

WITH RACHEL HOLTZMAN

PHOTOGRAPHY BY LIANNA TARANTIN
portraits by Caitlin Mitchell

ABRAMS, NEW YORK

EDITOR: Holly Dolce
DESIGNER: Deb Wood
PRODUCTION MANAGER:
   Denise LaCongo

LIBRARY OF CONGRESS
CONTROL NUMBER:
2018936278

ISBN: 978-1-4197-3473-1
B&N EDITION ISBN:
   978-1-4197-4025-1
EISBN: 978-1-68335-502-1

TEXT AND PHOTOGRAPHS
COPYRIGHT © 2019
SAKARA LIFE, INC.

JACKET AND COVER
© 2019 ABRAMS

PRINTED AND BOUND
IN THE UNITED STATES
10 9 8 7 6 5 4 3 2

*Abrams books are available
at special discounts when purchased
in quantity for premiums and
promotions as well as fundraising
or educational use. Special editions
can also be created to specification.
For details, contact specialsales@
abramsbooks.com or the address
below.*

*Abrams® is a registered trademark
of Harry N. Abrams, Inc.*

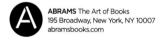

ABRAMS The Art of Books
195 Broadway, New York, NY 10007
abramsbooks.com

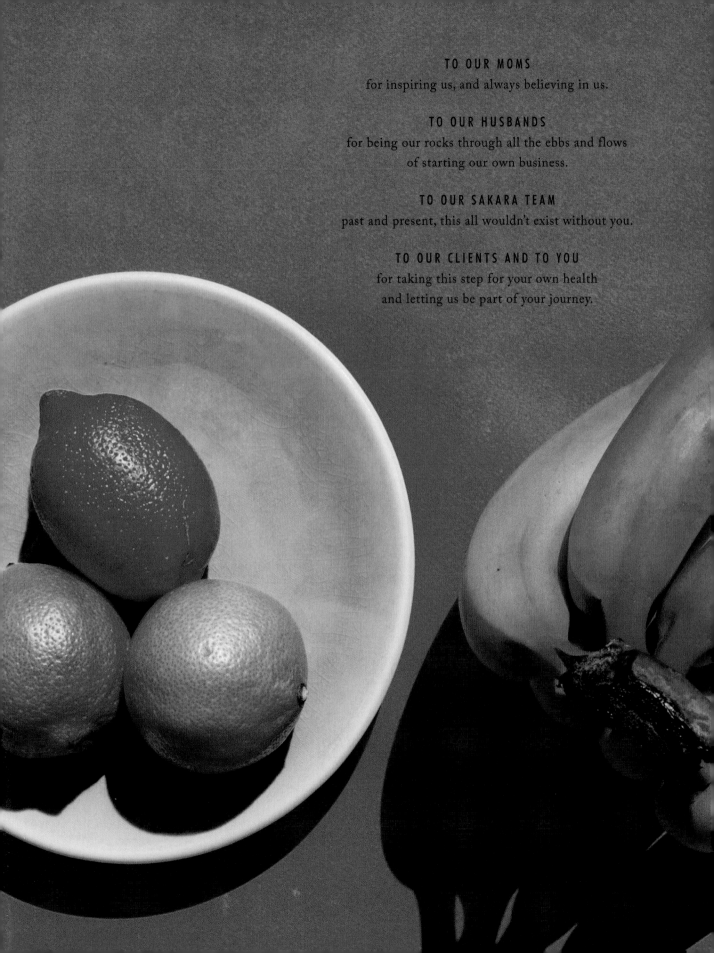

TO OUR MOMS
for inspiring us, and always believing in us.

TO OUR HUSBANDS
for being our rocks through all the ebbs and flows
of starting our own business.

TO OUR SAKARA TEAM
past and present, this all wouldn't exist without you.

TO OUR CLIENTS AND TO YOU
for taking this step for your own health
and letting us be part of your journey.

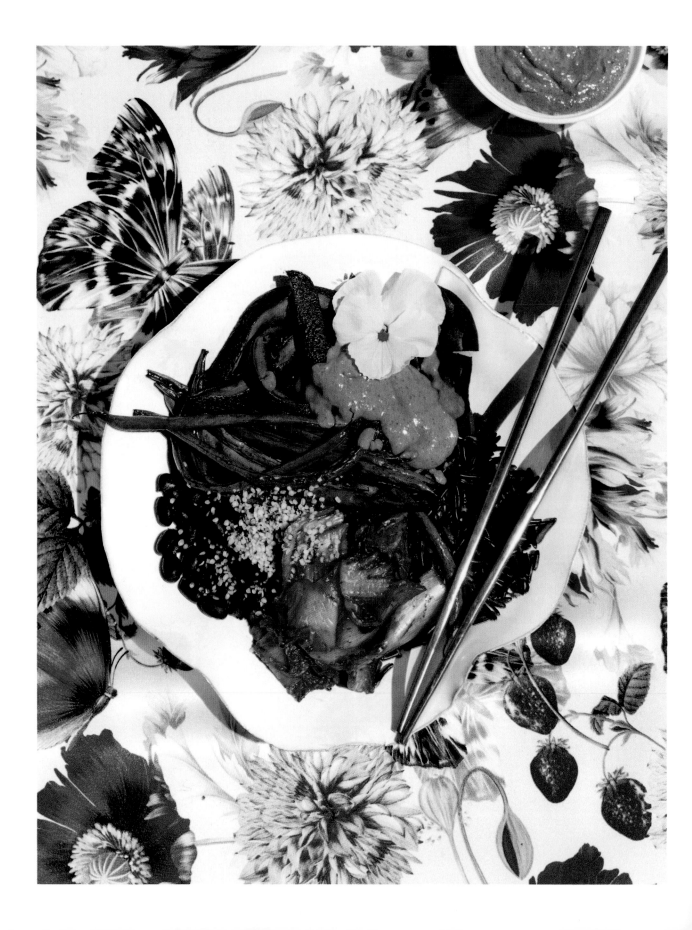

CONTENTS

"Food is one of the most powerful tools to help you manifest the things you want in life."

FOOD IS MEDICINE AND PLEASURE, and an incredibly potent catalyst for change. Once you realize that what you put into your body shapes every aspect of your life, food becomes your most important ally in feeling strong, smart, successful, sexy, seductive, sensual, sacred, and spiritual. For manifesting your dream life . . . your Sakara life.

Sakara didn't originally start out as a business, it started out as a solution to our own needs. We grew up as best friends in the small hippie-spiritual town of Sedona, Arizona, meditating, doing tai chi, making nut milks from scratch, and snacking on chlorella tablets that left our teeth stained dark green. We were surrounded by people who had come from all over the world seeking the curative power of Sedona's energy vortexes, psychics, and healers. Our community was a beautiful blend of out-of-the-box thinkers—New Agers, Buddhists, people who channeled aliens, and people who believed they were the descendants of wolves.

We like to think that the seed for starting Sakara was planted when we were about twelve, when we met. Whitney was the new girl in school, and we became fast friends from the moment we shared our first math class—as if our souls recognized each other. But, like all great journeys, it wasn't exactly a straight line from there to Sakara. After high school we parted ways for college, and while our paths eventually brought us back together in New York City, our relationships with health and healing had taken quite a detour.

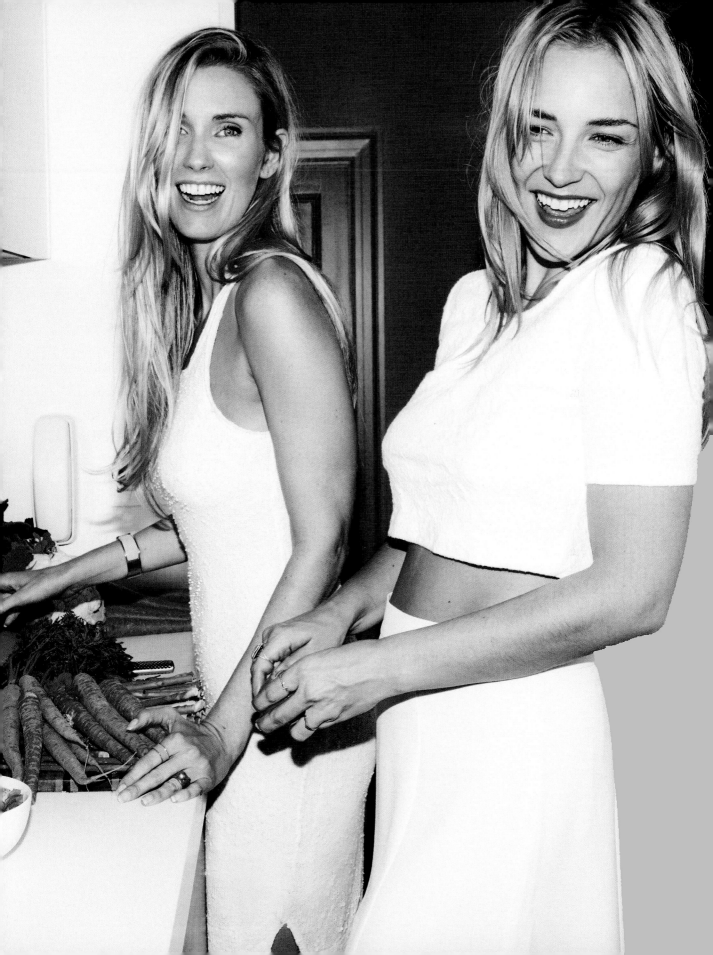

"I had to seek out the root cause of my symptoms— and treat that." WHITNEY TINGLE

I moved to New York to work on Wall Street at Merrill Lynch. I quickly fell into the typical corporate banker lifestyle of eighty-hour high-stress, low-sleep workweeks, punctuated by after-work drinks, quick, mindless meals, and bar food. Until, one morning, I woke up and realized I had gained fifteen pounds, and the cystic acne I had struggled with since high school was at an all-time worst. My face was covered in big painful cysts. It was affecting my career, my confidence, and my relationships.

WHITNEY'S STORY

By this point I had tried just about everything: all the "miracle treatments" I saw advertised on infomercials that promised perfect skin; crazy lights and laser treatments that peeled layers off my face and left me scabbed and scarred; different forms of hormone pills; and all the prescription treatments, from antibiotics (all the -cylines) to Z-Paks, the hard-core antibiotics given to obliterate pneumonia or bronchitis.

None of it worked. But I thought, *I'm in New York City, someone here has to be able to fix me!* I went to all the dermatologists I read about in magazines; doctor after doctor prescribed the same solution: Accutane, again. It has always been touted as the miracle drug for acne—and was, according to the doctors, my only option, even though I'd already tried it, without success. Along with the Accutane, I took Prozac because suicide is a possible side effect; had my blood tested every other week to make sure the Accutane wasn't damaging my liver; was put on birth control—and even signed a contract saying that if I got pregnant, I would have an abortion because of the high risk that the baby would come out with serious birth defects. I thought to myself, *If my body isn't a safe place for a baby, how can it be a safe place for me?* As I sat in the dermatologist's chair contemplating if I should do it and put my body at risk once again, a voice inside of me shouted, *DON'T DO IT. It's not the answer. Look inside and find the root cause, and treat that.*

When I was growing up, my mother was in and out of the hospital. Time and time again I'd see doctors seem to miraculously save her life. I knew that I wanted to be a healer too. So I moved to New York City to study premed, with a major in biochemistry. As part of the program I interned in a local hospital, shadowing a renowned cardiologist. I saw him save lives every day, but I also saw something else. Many of the patients he treated were suffering from things like heart disease, high blood pressure, high cholesterol, and diabetes—diseases that potentially could have been treated or prevented with the right lifestyle changes, if someone had intervened earlier and had given them recommendations for transforming their diets, exercise regimens, or mentalities. While I appreciated modern medicine and knew that it was helping to prolong these peoples' lives, this wasn't exactly the kind of healing I had had in mind. I felt that we were missing a step in helping people—what about the wellness *before* the illness? And how could I *keep* people well?

DANIELLE'S STORY

Meanwhile, I was in need of healing myself. I had been a chronic yo-yo dieter since I was nine years old. Food went from being something special that I shared with family and provided pleasure to being the enemy. I remember going to Costco with my mom and trying to sneak diet pills into the cart (I obviously got caught because Costco sells only about four thousand pills at a time, so they were pretty hard to hide). I tried every diet out there—Atkins, South Beach, even a diet where all I ate were fiber cookies I bought at the drugstore. I counted calories and carbs, perfectly portioned every meal, and got really good at saying no to food at the dinner table. I hid behind labels like "vegetarian" or "vegan" so I could tell people, "I can't eat that." Things got even more extreme when I was living in New York because I was putting myself through school by modeling and acting. I saw all the beautiful, thin women I was up against for jobs, which made me that much more resolved to deprive myself of anything that would keep me from my goals. I found new ways to avoid food, with cleanses and detoxes, until I was essentially subsisting on liquids.

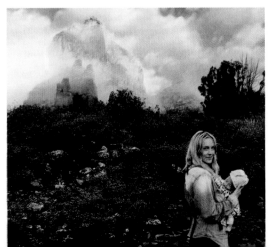

What ultimately brought us to our most grounded, balanced place was hitting our most unstable, unbalanced low—what we considered to be our rock bottom. Determined to cleanse her way back to health, Whitney was experimenting with the juice cleanses and detoxes that were just hitting the mainstream health world. And Danielle, who didn't need any excuse to try a new program, was happy to come along for the ride. We'd go to the Whole Foods in Tribeca and lug back huge bags of lemons with maple syrup and cayenne for the Master Cleanse. We did a candida cleanse where we were eating raw garlic (we had no friends during that time) and spoonfuls of coconut oil. Meanwhile, the day after a cleanse would end, Whitney would be back at the office, hustling hard, going out for drinks, and dipping into the calamari basket. As for Danielle, she took the cleanses to an even more restrictive level. She signed herself up for a twenty-one-day retreat in southern Arizona that would give her a new excuse to diet. It started with a seven-day water fast followed by two weeks of living off the land and learning to prepare (and eat) raw food meals, coupled with daily enemas and six hours of meditation. And she got sick. *Really* sick. Her body shut

OUR STORY

down—she could barely get out of bed, and making it up the tiny "hill" to get her meals felt like intense cardio. She couldn't digest her food properly, and her bloated stomach made her appear pregnant. She had a cough and a fever, and by the time she got home she looked so ill that Whitney took her straight to the hospital, where she was diagnosed with irritable bowel syndrome (i.e., "We have no idea what's wrong with your digestive system") and pneumonia (i.e., "Wow! I'm clearly willing to hurt myself to get the body I thought I had to have"). At that moment, something clicked in her brain. She had forgotten that food was nourishment—that it was there to make her feel better, not worse, and, more importantly, that it was the *solution* and not the problem.

That moment helped us see clearly how off-kilter we both were. We were both living at extremes, pushing boundaries in ways that were punishing our health. Then and there we decided to dedicate our lives to finding solutions to our wellness struggles, to seeking out the answers to these questions: What is true health? What does ultimate nutrition look like? And how can we make it a sustainable lifestyle? In Sedona, people understand the power of food as medicine and look to their plates

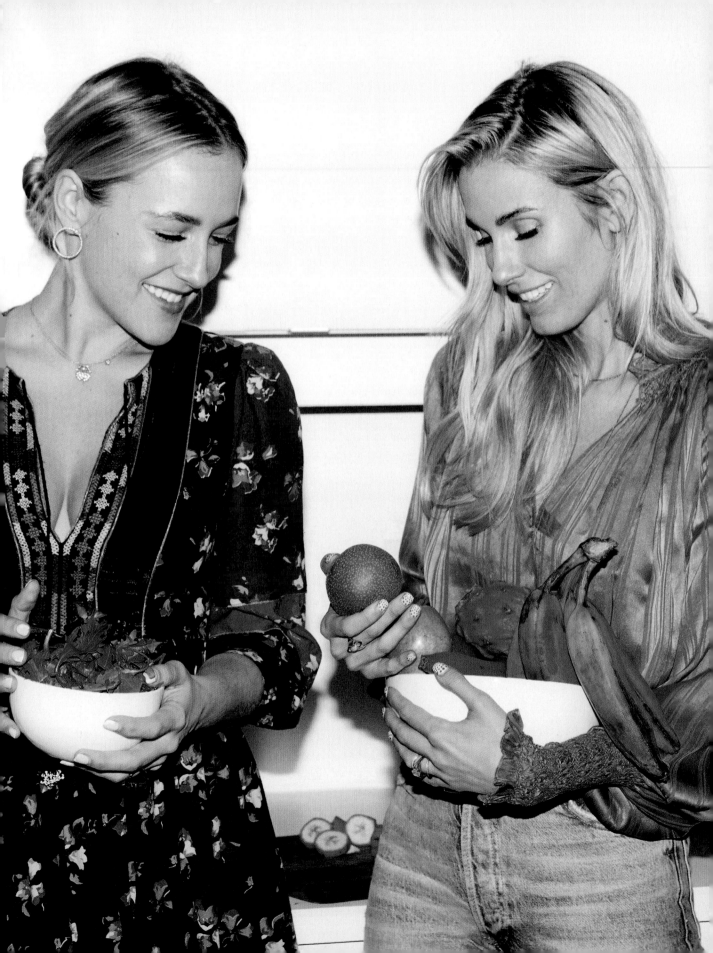

"I realized food is information. Diets never taught me that." DANIELLE DUBOISE

as the first step in the healing process. Somehow, we'd forgotten that along the way. But because we'd hit bottom, there was nowhere to go but up. Danielle decided she wanted to study nutrition instead of medicine, to heal herself but also to help others maintain their wellness—not just try to treat them once they've reached illness. We also started experimenting again, but this time in a different way.

We were no longer looking to food to help with acne or weight; we were using it as a tool to *build our health*. And we needed to start from scratch. No diet or cleanse had ever taken our well-being into consideration, so we set out to create a sustainable way of eating that did. We consulted Eastern and Western doctors, nutritionists, rabbis, shamans, Taoists, Ayurvedic gurus, and macrobiotic healers. We took the cutting-edge nutrition science Danielle was learning about in school (things like the importance of the microbiome and the study of nutrigenomics, or how what you eat determines which genes in your body are turned on or off or passed down from generation to generation) and paired it with the ancient food philosophies we had learned about growing up in Sedona—ones that cultures had been thriving on for thousands

of years. And we started to see the common threads that ran through them. These threads where modern science and ancient nutrition intersect became the pillars for us to live and eat by. We made these pearls of wisdom our guidelines (they would become Sakara's Pillars of Nutrition, which we'll talk about much more later in this book, page 20). Then we got in the kitchen and played. Using ourselves as guinea pigs, we created recipes that satisfied each of these guidelines, tinkering and testing until we got them right. And when we did, transformation is what we received. Within weeks, Danielle was able to eat with peace of mind and maintain her perfect weight without counting calories or grams of fat. She realized that she'd spent a lifetime worrying about eating too much, when she should really have been focused on eating enough of the right things. And Whitney was finally able to end her decade-long battle with acne. The redness and inflammation of her skin started subsiding, and she wasn't getting any new breakouts. She realized that she had been trying to treat her skin when she didn't have a skin issue—she had a *gut* issue. She saw the powerful connection between this control center in the body and matters such as mood, hormonal imbalance, and immune system strength. After years of obliterating the balance of bacteria in her gut with antibiotics, she was finally restoring the good flora and feeding it properly. Not only did her skin clear up, but things she didn't think were even related, such as her anxiety, also went away.

Once we experienced these major transformations, other people started to notice. Friends and neighbors could tell something was different—maybe it was our newfound glow, maybe it was confidence and wisdom, or maybe it was just the enormous bags of fruits and veggies they saw us lugging home from the farmers market every week. Anyway, they asked if we'd cook for them. So we did. We threw a dinner party, invited all our friends, and charged them for the meal. At the end of the night, we had seven hundred dollars—enough to register our business, buy a domain name, and invest in some marketing cards to hand out in cafés and yoga studios.

Every step of the way, our goal was to share the answers to the questions that we'd asked ourselves in Danielle's hospital room. Sakara was *the* answer to get us back to feeling like our best selves again, in our skin and in our hearts. And we made it our mission to

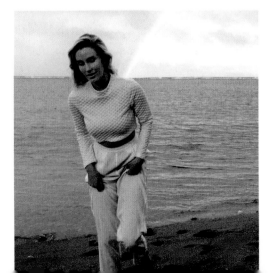

share that answer with the world. Today, we've delivered more than one million meals and have helped change the bodies—and lives—of thousands of people across the United States with our Sakara Life meal delivery program. Clients have reported clearer skin, more energy, healthy weight loss, better sleep, balanced moods, improved digestion, fewer cravings, and a stronger mind-body connection. They've even reported that our program has helped them with more serious conditions like Crohn's and colitis, and autoimmune disorders, including lupus and Hashimoto's. For some, we've been told it was their long-awaited solution for fertility issues, helping them conceive when they thought they never could. And it's helped others escape depression and reclaim their lives.

But Sakara is much more than a "meal delivery service"; it's a nutrition philosophy and a way of life. The meal delivery element is a tool—a convenient way to eat meals that follow that philosophy. And now we are finally happy to share some of our clients' favorite recipes from our signature program, so that you can make these meals and live the life too. We are so excited to be on this journey with you. Welcome to the Sakara Life.

Our
Sakara
Beliefs

WE BELIEVE in the power of PLANTS. That eating ORGANIC, whole, nutrient-rich foods can impact your health and your life.

WE BELIEVE you are what you do the majority of the time. In leafy greens, but also in MIMOSAS at Sunday brunch and in the joy of dark chocolate.

WE BELIEVE that FOOD should make you feel sexy. Body love, in the most delicious way possible.

WE BELIEVE in counting our BLESSINGS. Not points, carbs, or calories.

WE BELIEVE in making choices that will improve your quality of LIFE, not just your pants size. Although that will change too—trust us!

UNLOCK *Your* *Microbiome*

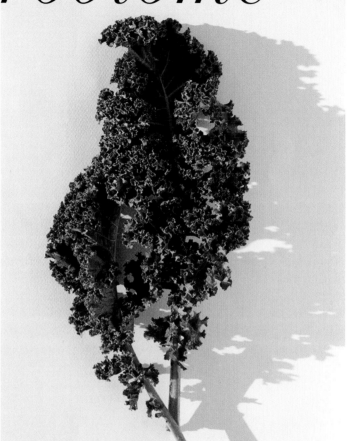

You may have heard the term *microbiome* thrown around—especially by us, because we talk about it *all the time*. It sounds big and scary, but what it refers to is the ecosystem of microbes living in and on your body. In this book, we're mainly interested in the six pounds (2.7 kg) of flora living in your gut, or digestive system. And we're bringing up the microbiome, yet again, because it is one of *the* most important aspects of health, and most certainly the future of nutrition. *Every single one* of the Sakara pillars leads back to this power center because your microbiome isn't a static element. It's ever changing—for better or for worse. We like to think of this group of microbes as your little pets: You need to keep them fed and watered and loved. And, in return, they will love you back.

HERE ARE THE THREE BASIC THINGS YOU NEED TO KNOW:

1

THE BACTERIA IN YOUR BELLY ARE CALLING ALL THE SHOTS.

Seventy percent of the cells that make up your immune system live in your gut, and 90 percent of your serotonin is made there, not in your brain. So your microbiome isn't in charge only of digesting food; it also has a hand in how well your body can detoxify and defend itself from illness, in hormone production and sex drive, and in your mood. An unhappy gut can lead to just about anything from digestive issues (such as bloating, gas, or constipation) to skin conditions (such as acne and eczema), anxiety and depression, and suppressed immunity or even autoimmune disease.

2

YOUR GUT AFFECTS YOUR FOOD.

Living the Sakara Life is all about balance, so we fully support the occasional indulgence and recognize that it's not just inevitable but necessary! When your gut is cared for and thriving, and your body is firing on all cylinders, it can handle the occasional truffle fry or martini. The Sakara lifestyle changes how the body assimilates foods that aren't healing, easing reactions like bloating and inflammation, and even affecting how the body uses the non-nourishing calories. In fact, the better you eat (i.e., plenty of leafy greens, colorful plants, and healthy fats), the smarter your body gets and the more efficient a machine it becomes, knowing exactly how much energy it needs to use to function at its best.

3

YOUR FOOD AFFECTS YOUR GUT.

So what do all those essential, life-giving, body-balancing bacteria eat? Plants! A diet rich in fiber-packed whole foods feeds the good guys and helps them multiply and diversify—essential for maintaining robust gut health. What's good for you is also good for your gut, and, as we like to say, treat your gut well, and it will treat you well.

THE SAKARA
Philosophy

THE 9 PILLARS OF NUTRITION

In a (raw, organic) nutshell, the Sakara approach to transformational eating is based on a whole-food, plant-rich diet that includes fresh, nutrient-dense, and delicious ingredients. We don't count calories, carbs, points, or pounds. We're not vegans, vegetarians, raw foodists, or extremists in any way. We simply believe in fresh meals, prepared with loving hands, using the healthiest, most hydrating and nourishing ingredients possible.

Sakara is built on the idea that food is the foundation for change—change in your physical body and also in your mental state, your life force energy, and your ability to manifest the things you want in the world—all without giving up the things you love to eat and do. Through years of research and testing, these simple, seemingly universal truths became Sakara's guidelines, or what we call our Pillars of Nutrition, and the nutrition foundation for each of our nourishing recipes.

"Food is a tool to get you to your ultimate desired outcome in life: fulfilling your purpose on this planet. Living your life to the fullest and becoming the fullest expression of yourself. You cannot do this if your physical body, the vessel that carries you around in the world, isn't functioning properly. That is why food is the place we start. Because so many of us are moving around in a vehicle that is not functioning at peak performance, and that is something we can change."

COUNT BLESSINGS, *NOT* CALORIES

1.

A calorie is a measurement, not a nutrient.

A calorie is used to measure energy in a fixed system, meaning it does not take into account the actual nutrition of your food or how your body (not a fixed system!) handles that food. We can promise you that building your best body does not involve counting calories!

Food is not made up solely of calories. According to Mark Hyman, MD, best-selling author and director of Cleveland Clinic's Center for Functional Medicine, "Some calories are addictive, others healing, some fattening, some metabolism-boosting." Why? "Because food doesn't just contain calories, it contains *information*. Every bite of food you eat broadcasts a set of coded instructions to your body—instructions that can create either health or disease."

A healthy microbiome—the community of bacteria that lives in and on your body, which we discussed on page 18—also makes a big difference in the nutrients and energy we can extract from our food. Recent research has shown that a flourishing microbiome in the digestive tract is going to be more efficient at breaking down your food and putting it to use as energy. And eating a plant-based, organic diet is the number-one thing you can do to promote a healthy gut microbiome.

So instead of fixating on counting calories, we focus on getting enough minerals, vitamins, antioxidants, fibers, and hydration from our food—something that naturally happens when you follow these pillars and that will lead to your looking and feeling like your best self.

2.

T hat's the biggest question anyone who has eaten a plant-based diet, let alone ordered a vegetarian salad at dinner, is bombarded with. Thanks to political lobbying, corporate advertising, and misleading information pretty much everywhere about how much protein we actually need, many people see plant-based eaters as malnourished hippies who survive on rabbit food, grass, and love. It's not true. According to a study published in *JAMA: The Journal of the American Medical Association*, we need to aim for only .36 grams of protein per pound (.5 kg) of body weight a day. That's it! In other words, a person weighing 150 pounds (68 kg) would need only about 54 grams of daily protein. Did you know that four cups (270 g) of kale packs 12 grams of protein? And a cup (165 g) of chickpeas has 15 grams of protein? Make yourself a simple yet delicious kale salad with chickpeas or hummus and that's half your needed protein for the day.

Science break: Protein is composed of twenty amino acids, eleven of which your body produces naturally and nine of which you can obtain only through food sources. The term *complete protein* refers to a food that has all these amazing amino acids—you'll find many complete proteins in the plant world. There are plenty of plant-based sources that provide complete protein for the body (e.g., nuts like walnuts, almonds, macadamia, and cashews; seeds like pumpkin seeds, sunflower seeds, and sesame seeds; beans like chickpeas, black beans, and lentils; and even some things you might not expect, like goji berries and cauliflower!). The human body is amazingly adept at utilizing its resources, pulling the amino acids it needs over the course of a few days to form complete proteins. We believe if you want to eat things other than plants responsibly, that's okay too. As long as you're eating a healthy variety of plants in a large enough quantity (think abundance!), you shouldn't need to stress over protein.

STOP STRESSING ABOUT PROTEIN

"But where do you get your protein?!"

EAT YOUR WATER

The true fountain of youth.

Hydration is *everything*. Literally! Your body is 60 to 80 percent water, and every cell, organ, and bit of tissue needs water to function optimally—not to mention look and feel supple and fresh. And one of the best ways to deliver all that essential H_2O to your body is to eat your water by consuming whole, fresh foods, which are packed with their own natural hydration systems.

While drinking water is an essential part of the detoxification process, when you eat fruits and vegetables—most of which are more than 90 percent water!—you're not only delivering ample hydration to your cells, you're also getting microbiome-friendly fiber, age-fighting antioxidants and phytochemicals, and health-preserving vitamins and minerals while leaving your insides, as well as your skin, supple and glowing. We like to say that our favorite beauty products aren't what we put on our faces; they're what we put in our bodies.

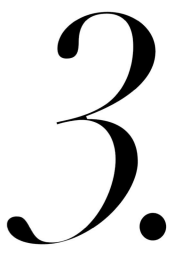

3.

EAT MORE GREENS THAN YOU EVER IMAGINED

*Greens are a foundational element in the
Sakara Life nutritional philosophy.*

If you only take away one message from this book, let it be this: Eat more greens. Not only are greens filled with microbiome-supporting fiber, lots of hydration, and amino acids for protein, they're packed with chlorophyll (it's what gives them their green color), which is known to support detoxification and oxygenate the body. When it comes to one of the most important foods in your arsenal, we think integrative gastroenterologist, microbiome expert, and bestselling author Robynne Chutkan, MD, put it best: "Greens are the least consumed food in the standard American diet, yet they're the most essential for inner and outer health. They come the closest of any food to meeting our ideal nutritional requirements. If you want to encourage the growth of good bacteria, heal inflammation, improve motility, crowd out parasites, eliminate yeast, get rid of belly fat, dissolve gallstones, balance your pH, quiet down your irritable bowel syndrome (IBS), prevent diverticulitis, cut your risk of colon cancer in half, boost your energy, banish your bloat, and really glow, then the single most important thing you can do is eat greens every single day." Enough said? That's why we recommend—and our meals provide—six to eight cups (400 to 540 g) of greens every day. It might be more greens than you ever imagined, but this little secret will change your life. And as Dr. Chutkan says, "You don't have to like them, you just have to eat them."

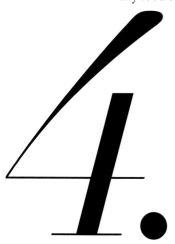

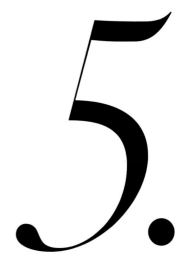

In the 1980s and '90s, the world turned against fat. The party line was that fat was what was making us fat, and that low-fat or fat-free foods filled with starches, sugars, salts, and artificial ingredients were the key to an optimal weight and health. Fortunately, science caught up.

Healthy fats—or fats that come from whole-plant sources, such as cold-pressed olive oil, avocados, coconuts, and nuts—are a Sakara power ingredient that we use in all of our recipes. They are key to keeping you energized, focused, lean, and radiant. They are essential for digestion, helping the body to absorb fat-soluble nutrients and keep things moving during the digestive process. They are harder for your body to break down, so they keep you full, and your metabolism stoked, longer. They contribute to building stronger hair, skin, and nails. And they help both to reduce oxidative stress in the brain and to enhance the synaptic connections among neurons for better memory, learning, and clarity. Oh, and did we mention they're delicious? You won't find a Sakara meal without a dollop, schmear, or drizzle of luscious, decadent fatty goodness.

Fat is one of the body's most basic building blocks.

MAKE PEACE WITH *FATS*

EAT THE RAINBOW

We believe that food should be bright, vibrant, and beautiful (like you!).

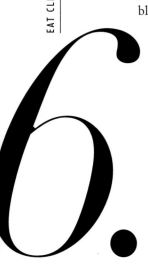

That's not just because it makes for a sexier plate of food but also because the colors of the plant rainbow are code for a unique set of vitamins, minerals, nutrients, and antioxidants to nourish your body from the inside out. The more colors you eat, the wider the array of nutrients with which you are fueling your body. According to skin whisperer Nicholas Perricone, MD, "Plant pigments don't just add color to fruits and vegetables, they also serve as the top dietary sources of antiaging antioxidants and disease-preventative phytonutrients." These phytonutrients are nature's best anti-inflammatory agents, helping the body repair damage from everyday wear and tear, reverse or prevent disease, and preserve vitality. These are nutrients your body needs and can *only* get from plants. As a general rule, in every meal you eat, try to get at least three to five different colors on your plate to make sure you're filling your body with all the healthy love it needs.

In order to give our bodies the fuel they need to function at their best, we must strive to eat foods high in essential nutrients—especially the ones that our bodies can't make themselves. One of the best ways to tell whether a food should have a place in your rotation is to consider its *nutrient density*. Scientifically speaking, nutrient-dense foods are those that have an extremely high nutrient-to-size ratio.

To provide another nutrient boost to our meals, we like adding at least one "superfood," or a plant that is particularly packed with disease-fighting, health-promoting power. Because of modern farming practices and environmental changes, our soil doesn't contain the nutrients it once did, meaning our fruits and vegetables don't always contain the nutrients they once did. So we have to make an extra effort to ensure that we're getting all the vitamins, minerals, and nutrition that our bodies need. Superfoods like hemp and chia seeds, miso, turmeric, spirulina, and cacao have been called upon for centuries in traditional healing practices, and today continue to help maximize the nutrients in your diet and deliver nourishing compounds that you might not otherwise be getting. We like adding superfoods to pretty much anything we're eating, sprinkling them over salads or blending them into dressings.

Superfoods equal super you.

PACK ON THE NUTRIENTS

SULFUR
IS BEAUTIFUL

*You'll never look at a cruciferous vegetable
in the same way again.*

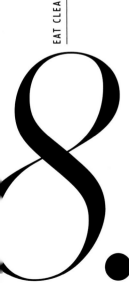

Sulfur is one of the most beneficial minerals in the body, assisting its systems in fighting off bacteria and flushing out toxins. According to Terry Wahls, MD, author of *The Wahls Protocol* who used food to help treat her own autoimmune disease, "Sulfur has been used medicinally for centuries to treat infections, tumors, and health problems related to blood vessels." In her research, she has found that sulfur "nourishes mitochondria, removes toxins from cells, and helps create proteins and connective tissue necessary for joint, skin, and blood vessel health." While sulfur may not be the first nutrient you think of when you hear the term *beauty food*, it plays an integral role in both detoxification (which helps your skin look dewy and fresh) and in building shiny, strong hair and nails. Sulfur is also a precursor to glutathione, one of the most powerful antiaging antioxidants. This is why you'll find plenty of sulfurous veggies like kale, Brussels sprouts, broccoli, cauliflower, and cabbage on our plates.

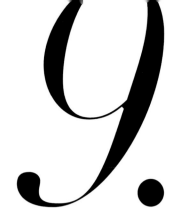

Everything we've been talking about thus far has been leading up to this ultimate piece of our nutritional philosophy: The body is wise. It knows how to digest, it knows how to cleanse. It knows how to protect itself, and to eliminate what it doesn't need. It also knows what it does need and, most importantly, how to communicate that to you—as long as you know how to listen.

Unfortunately, there are a lot of things that stand in the way of true body intelligence and mess with the signals that your body is sending you—namely, processed foods, refined sugar, chemical additives and preservatives, and even stress and some medications. These things change your body's natural signals—I'm hungry, I'm full, I'm tired, I'm happy—and are endocrine or hormone disruptors.

But when you let go of the foods that are hijacking your brain or giving your body the wrong information and embrace the foods your body inherently knows how to use, you will be able to connect with its purest, most honest voice. You won't need to count calories or rely on nutrition facts labels to be aware if something is "good" or how much to eat, because your body will tell you what it genuinely wants and genuinely needs. It will let you know when it's hungry and when it's full. It will let you know when it is feeling robust and strong, and when it needs a little extra tenderness. So long as you're feeding your body the food it needs to thrive, your gut will be your truest guide. And when you are able to listen and trust your gut, it will lead you to manifest your deepest desires. The desires that are aligned with the life you truly want to live. And that is a beautiful thing.

The body is wise.

TRUST YOUR GUT

EAT CLEAN, *Play DIRTY*

We don't believe in restriction, and we definitely don't believe in guilt. Instead, you'll find us lighting a candle at the altar of *balance*. That's an essential component of living life to the fullest—of experiencing bliss! Sometimes "balance" means having that glass of wine or ordering the scone instead of the green smoothie. The Sakara motto is: "**Eat clean, play dirty**," because taking good care of yourself in a long-term, sustainable way is as much about pleasure and the freedom to make choices that feel good as it is about nourishing your body. To us, true health isn't all buttoned-up and polished. It's a little imperfect—and that's kind of perfect.

THE BASICS

When starting the Sakara program, clients often ask us, "What foods should I avoid?"

We get it. Give us a rule, and we'll follow it. And we get it: You want results. So here's what we suggest: Try one of our breakfasts every day. Make any meal a lunch or a dinner. Stick to a single portion. Enjoy the occasional dessert or cocktail (or both). Our philosophy is that eating what you need to be eating every day is the foundation for true health. When you do that, you'll not only check off all the boxes for foods that your body thrives on but also innately crowd out some of the foods that aren't as kind to your systems. You'll also begin to change on the cellular level. By eating lots of leafy greens and other colorful veggies, you'll develop a taste for those flavors. You'll also turn your body into a flora-powered digestion machine, so if on occasion you do happen to eat foods that are less than ideal, your systems are better equipped to handle them, with fewer negative side effects.

Each of the recipes in this book follows our Pillars of Nutrition and embraces the same spirit of plenty. The foods you'll see called for in abundance include vegetables, fruits, nuts, seeds, legumes, leafy greens, fresh high-quality cold-pressed fats (such as extra-virgin olive, avocado, and coconut oil), natural probiotics (fermented foods such as kimchi and sauerkraut), and functional, nutrient-dense superfoods (such as hemp seeds, chia seeds, turmeric, and spirulina).

But while we would never want to come between you and a guilty pleasure, there are some foods and food additives that are particularly damaging. When it comes to foods we avoid, go with this: If it's not made by Mother Nature, it's not made for us to eat. Highly processed foods, hydrogenated oils, corn syrup, artificial colors, preservatives, bromates, and genetically modified produce are on the "try to avoid" list. We choose to focus on quality instead, eating organic and limiting the amounts of toxins that enter our bodies as best we can (with a little leeway for life). While we don't think you need to be a vegan in order to reach your ultimate wellness, we do think it's important to make sure you're getting enough plants in your diet, and when choosing animal products, you do so with mindfulness and moderation. These foods should be selected with the same standards you would use when sourcing plants—ideally organic and raised close to where you live. And be aware of how much of these foods you're inviting into your diet—it's easy to make meat and cheese (along with bread, coffee, and alcohol) staples in our diet if we're not conscious and careful.

> **TRY ONE OF OUR BREAKFASTS EVERY DAY. MAKE ANY MEAL A LUNCH OR A DINNER. STICK TO A SINGLE PORTION. ENJOY THE OCCASIONAL DESSERT OR COCKTAIL (OR BOTH).**

A DAY IN THE SAKARA LIFE

WAKE UP

To gently awaken your body, enjoy a glass of warm lemon water (or a glass of water with our Beauty Water Concentrate), and, as you're drinking, think of three things you are thankful for (we suggest writing them down and taking the list with you to remind you of all the blessings that fill your life!).

BREAKFAST

If possible (and we say anything is *always* possible), wake up early enough so that you are able to enjoy your first meal of the day at your kitchen table *without* the TV on and with your e-mail *closed*. Eating while stressed can slow down your digestive system, which taxes the entire body. Conscious eating, on the other hand, leads to conscious living! If you like to exercise in the morning, save your breakfast for after your sweat session.

MID-MORNING (and also mid-afternoon)

Stay hydrated with lots of lemon or lime water or tea. Try any of our current blends: Detox, Digestive, or Youth + Beauty.

LUNCH

Try to pause to enjoy your midday meal. If you can get away, step out of the office for a moment and breathe some fresh air. Take some time for your food and for yourself.

Eat slowly and chew well, which not only helps ease the digestion process but also gives your brain time to register that your body is full.

DINNER

Try to eat dinner on the earlier side (at least two hours before you go to bed), so that your body is focusing on restoring itself as you sleep, not digesting your last meal. Remember to eat thoughtfully and chew your food slowly and thoroughly. Finish off the night with another cup of herbal tea or a glass of water with Sakara Detox Water Concentrate, if you enjoy something soothing before bed. Tomorrow is a whole new beautiful day for you to take charge.

AS FOR SNACKING

As you live the Sakara Life, you'll notice that you don't feel the need to snack as often as you used to. That's because you're getting all the nutrients, water, fiber, and fats you need, so your body is content and full of the good stuff. But you may also notice that from time to time you're hungry between meals. Allowing yourself to be a little hungry every now and then offers your body a great chance to direct some of its vital energy toward healing itself, rather than constantly sending that blood and other resources to your stomach and digestive system. Digestion taxes your body's energy stores, so when you give your body some downtime between meals, your digestive system gets a well-deserved break. And by letting yourself experience hunger between meals, you're helping to reset your natural hunger point as well, meaning you can see how much food your body actually *needs* to eat, as opposed to how much it has grown accustomed to eating.

That said, snacking is not a bad thing! If you're truly hungry, eat. If drinking some extra water or tea doesn't do the trick, have some raw fruits or veggies, which are easily digested snacks that are high in fiber and water content, so they will support the eliminating functions of your body.

YOUR DAILY GREENS

Eating leafy greens, and plenty of them (we recommend six to eight cups, or 400 to 540 grams, daily!), is one of the main pillars of the Sakara Life nutritional philosophy, which is why most of our recipes call for a healthy dose of these chlorophyll-packed goods. But in the case of dishes that aren't particularly leafy (wraps, soups, sandwiches, pizzas), we recommend adding a hit of Daily Greens: three to four cups (200 to 270 g) of cooked or raw greens. Keep it simple by tossing together your favorite mix with lemon juice and olive oil, or go for glory with one of our favorite dressings (pages 201–204) plus a sprinkling of seeds or nuts; or lightly steam or sauté the greens with plenty of garlic and a drizzle of olive oil.

MOVE IT

Daily movement is an integral part of the Sakara lifestyle—it's cleansing and fat-burning, and, if done correctly, will send your spirits soaring. Exercising is a great way to eliminate toxins because it activates the lymphatic system and encourages elimination through the colon, lungs, and skin. Pick an activity that gets you outside or involves a loved one so that you can nourish more than just your body. And don't be afraid to get physical and intimate with your body—learn to love it, respect it, and be its number-one advocate.

PUTTING IT ALL TOGETHER

We realize that this is a lot of new information to sort through, and that it might seem like overload for just a few healthy meals. But we promise you that the Sakara journey is about so much more. By creating a robust foundation with fresh, whole plants, and with your mind and body in solidarity, you'll be able to unlock your goals and dreams. You'll be well on your way to living the life you've always envisioned for yourself. Ultimately, this transformation is about claiming true happiness—in what you eat, in how your body feels, and in the thoughts that drift through your mind. So go forth, unleash, unfurl, and unfold. And, every now and then, remember to get a little *dirty*.

NOW, GET COOKING

Here is what we suggest keeping in mind as you cook your way through the book.

ALWAYS CHOOSE ORGANIC. That goes for produce *and* dry goods.

IT'S OKAY TO TAKE A SHORTCUT! Buy prechopped or spiralized veggies (organic), or canned beans (organic, from BPA-free containers)—we won't judge.

WORK AHEAD TO SAVE TIME. Prepare recipe staples like rice, quinoa, or beans (if you prefer the ritual of cooking them versus popping open a can) and store them in containers. Peel or chop your veggies. Assemble wraps and bowls and shake up a couple of dressings.

DON'T WASH YOUR PRODUCE until you're ready to use it. A great excuse to be a little lazy! Washing produce before storing it adds moisture, which encourages spoilage. Wrap leafy greens loosely in dishcloths or paper towels to keep them dry and fresh. When it's time to cook, use an organic veggie wash to clean your produce, or make your own by mixing one part vinegar to three parts water.

USE FILTERED WATER in recipes wherever possible. Clean water is just as important as clean food!

THINK PINK. Himalayan salt, that is. Unlike highly processed table salt, which is stripped of all but one mineral (sodium) and can contain bleaching and anticaking agents, plus traces of aluminum, Himalayan salt contains more than eighty-four minerals and trace elements including calcium, magnesium, potassium, copper, and iron. If you can't find it in your local store and would prefer not to buy it online, opt for sea salt.

FREESTYLE! Don't feel that you have to follow each recipe to a T. If you can't find a specific ingredient, make the recipe your own by adding veggies left over from another recipe, swapping the sauce, or adjusting the spice level. Play and explore!

MAKE COOKING A CEREMONY OF SELF-LOVE. Take in the smells and sounds. Embrace the process and learning new recipes and techniques. Enjoy the fact that you're doing something *really, truly good* for your body. Be fully present as you prepare your meals, and send gratitude to the food and every hand that touched it along the way—from the farmer's to your own.

THE SAKARA BLESSING

*Before enjoying a meal—even if you're eating while sitting at your desk—
share this blessing to tap into the vibrational frequency of your food:*

Bless this food
and let it nourish my body.
Gratitude for all the hands
that touched it and
allowed it to be on my plate.
Bless the earth for providing me
with everything I need to be
healthy, happy,
and free.

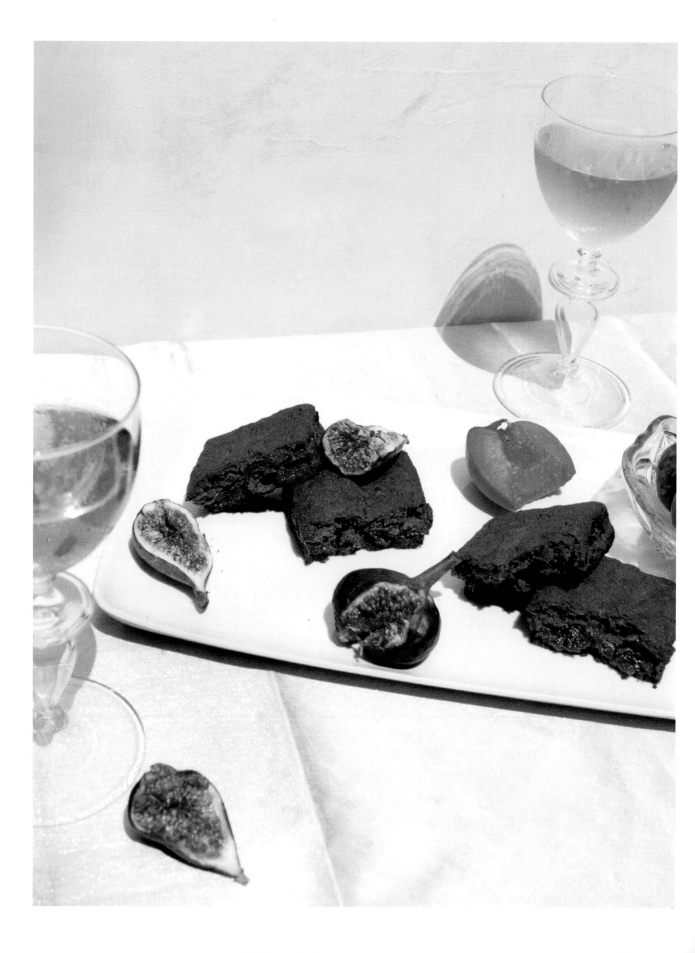

Breakfast should be enjoyable. Something to entice you out of bed and start your day right—nutrient-dense foods that give you energy, rev your metabolism, and lay the foundation for a very sweet day.

DETOX TEA APRICOT-FIG BARS, *following page*

DETOX TEA APRICOT-FIG BARS

MAKES 10 TO 12 BARS

FOR THE DOUGH

3 tea bags of Sakara Detox Tea, rooibos tea, or hibiscus tea, or 3 teaspoons loose tea

1 tablespoon chia seeds

1 cup (90 g) oat flour

¼ cup (50 g) coconut palm sugar

¼ teaspoon baking soda

⅛ teaspoon Himalayan salt

1 teaspoon ground cinnamon

¼ teaspoon ground cardamom

¼ cup (60 ml) plus 1 tablespoon coconut oil

1 tablespoon wildflower honey

1 teaspoon pure vanilla extract

FOR THE FIG FILLING

½ cup (75 g) dried figs, roughly chopped

½ cup (100 g) dried apricots, roughly chopped

2 teaspoons fresh lemon juice

Pinch of Himalayan salt

½ vanilla bean

You deserve to look and feel your absolute best in life—to be light, bright, and glowing and to release toxins that are weighing you down so your spirit can soar. When we formulated our Sakara Detox Tea, our intention was to help you truly shine with a special blend of digestion-supporting, metabolism-stoking roots, grasses, and flowers. The tea also helps to hydrate your body and reduce hunger between meals, allowing your body to reset.

These cardamom-perfumed bars are infused with the healing plants we put into our signature tea: red rooibos, a tea variety from South Africa that's rich in age-fighting antioxidants and fat-fighting compounds; lemongrass, a citrus-flavored medicinal plant known to detoxify the digestive tract, liver, kidneys, bladder, and pancreas by flushing toxins out of the body; and rose, which helps calm the adrenal system while soothing the senses with its delicate floral flavor and aroma.

If you don't have our tea, feel free to substitute a high-quality rooibos tea or hibiscus tea, which, in addition to having a gorgeous deep-blush color, is a healing agent. These can help lower blood pressure, reduce oxidative stress, keep blood sugar levels stable, and elevate mood.

1   Make the dough: In a large mug, add 1 cup (240 ml) of boiling water to the tea. Let steep for 10 minutes.

2   In a small bowl, whisk together the chia seeds and 3 tablespoons of the tea. Reserve the remaining tea for the filling. Set the mixture aside to gel for 10 minutes.

3   In a food processor, combine the flour, sugar, baking soda, salt, cinnamon, and cardamom and pulse just to mix. Add the oil, honey, vanilla, and chia-tea gel and pulse until the mixture forms a ball. Turn out the dough onto a sheet of plastic wrap. Wrap the dough tightly and form it into a disk. Chill it in the fridge for at least 1 hour or overnight.

4   Make the filling: In a small saucepan, combine the figs, apricots, lemon juice, and salt with ½ cup (120 ml) of the reserved tea over medium-low heat. Scrape the vanilla seeds into the pot and toss in the pod too. Bring to a gentle simmer and cook until the figs and apricots start to soften and the mixture thickens, 10 to 15 minutes. Remove the pot from the heat and carefully fish out the vanilla pod and discard. Transfer the mixture to a food processor and pulse until the mixture is slightly chunky.

5   Assemble the bars: Preheat the oven to 350°F (175°C). Line a baking sheet with parchment paper and set aside.

6   Unwrap the chilled dough from the plastic and place it on a piece of parchment paper. Lay another sheet of parchment paper on top and use a rolling pin to roll out the dough until it is roughly a 4 by 11-inch (10 by 28 cm) rectangle and about ¼ inch (6 mm) thick. Spread the fig and apricot filling evenly over the dough. Using the edge of the parchment to help, gently lift one of the long edges of the rectangle and fold it over the filling (as though you're folding a letter). Repeat with the second side and press lightly to seal. Slice the rectangle into 1-inch (2.5 cm) pieces and arrange them seam side down on the prepared baking sheet.

7   Bake the bars for 15 to 20 minutes, or until the dough is just turning golden brown. Let the bars cool completely before storing at room temperature for up to 3 days.

Light WORK

FIND YOUR WHY Set an intention when starting your recipes. Remind yourself why making and eating these foods are important to you. Is there something you're looking to change, grow, manifest? Get down to the root cause of what it is. If you want to lose a few pounds (we don't judge), have more energy, heal from something you've been battling with—get down to the why behind it. What in your life do you believe will change if you achieve your goal? Will you be happier? Will you try something new? Start a new job? Find love? Be loved? Whatever it is, see if you can visualize it actually happening now. And as you eat each meal, feel yourself getting closer to that desired place. That life you want. And start to take the steps to make it happen.

39

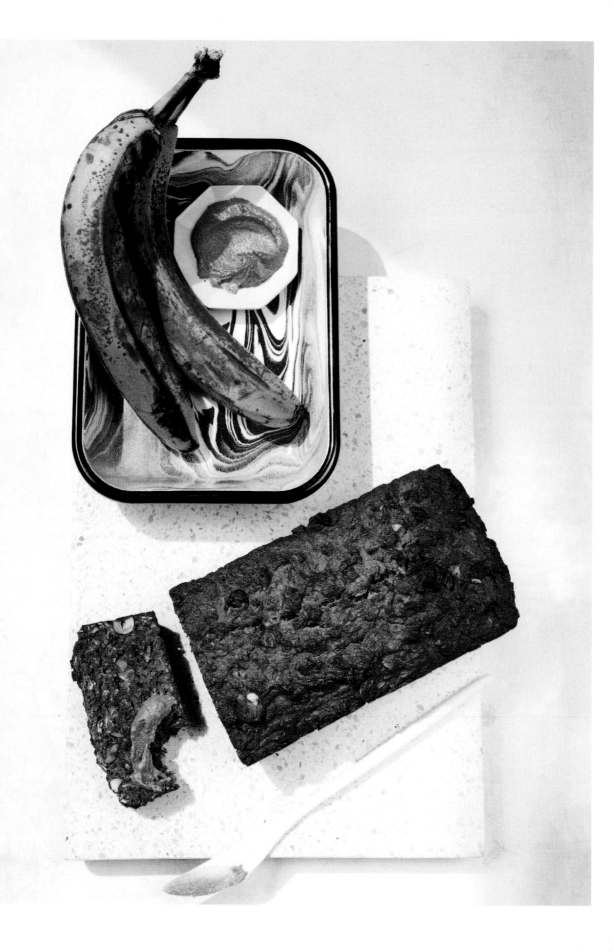

CLASSIC BANANA BREAD WITH VANILLA-TAHINI BUTTER

**MAKES 1 LOAF
(ABOUT 12 SLICES)**

FOR THE BANANA BREAD

1 tablespoon flaxseed meal

3 tablespoons extra-virgin coconut oil, melted, plus more for the pan

3 medium-ripe bananas, mashed (about 1½ cups/ 350 g)

½ teaspoon pure vanilla extract

½ cup (95 g) coconut palm sugar

3 tablespoons raw honey

3½ teaspoons baking powder

¾ teaspoon sea salt

½ teaspoon ground cinnamon

1¼ cups (120 g) almond meal

1½ cups (135 g) oat flour

1¼ cups (112 g) gluten-free oats

¾ cup (105 g) almonds, finely chopped

1 cup (135 g) hazelnuts, finely chopped

FOR THE VANILLA-TAHINI BUTTER

1 cup (240 ml) store-bought organic pumpkin puree

1 cup (240 ml) tahini

2 tablespoons wildflower honey

½ teaspoon pure vanilla extract

Himalayan salt

Banana bread is a soul-soothing food, so we came up with a plant-based, gluten-free, dairy-free version that trades processed flour and sugar for protein-dense oats, almond meal, coconut palm sugar and raw honey, and chopped nuts. To make it even more decadent, we've added a velvety spread that's the perfect combination of mineral- and vitamin-rich tahini and antioxidant-packed squash.

1   Make the banana bread: In a small bowl, stir together the flaxseed meal with 2 tablespoons of water. Allow the mixture to sit for 2 minutes to thicken slightly.

2   Preheat the oven to 350°F (175°C). Lightly grease an 8 by 4½-inch (20 by 11 cm) loaf pan with oil and set aside.

3   In a large bowl, whisk together the bananas, vanilla, oil, sugar, honey, baking powder, salt, cinnamon, and flaxseed meal–water mixture. Add the almond meal, flour, and oats and stir until combined. Fold in the almonds and hazelnuts.

4   Pour the batter into the prepared loaf pan and bake for 1 hour, or until the bread feels firm and the top has turned golden brown and is slightly cracked. If the bread starts to brown too quickly, cover with foil and continue baking.

5   Make the vanilla-tahini butter: In a food processor or blender, combine the pumpkin, tahini, honey, and vanilla with a pinch of salt and blend until smooth.

6   Enjoy the bread warm, slathered with the tahini butter and a tiny sprinkle of salt. Store leftovers in the fridge—the bread for up to 3 days, the tahini for up to 5. This bread also freezes well: Wrap the loaf in foil and a freezer-safe plastic bag and store in the freezer for up to 2 months.

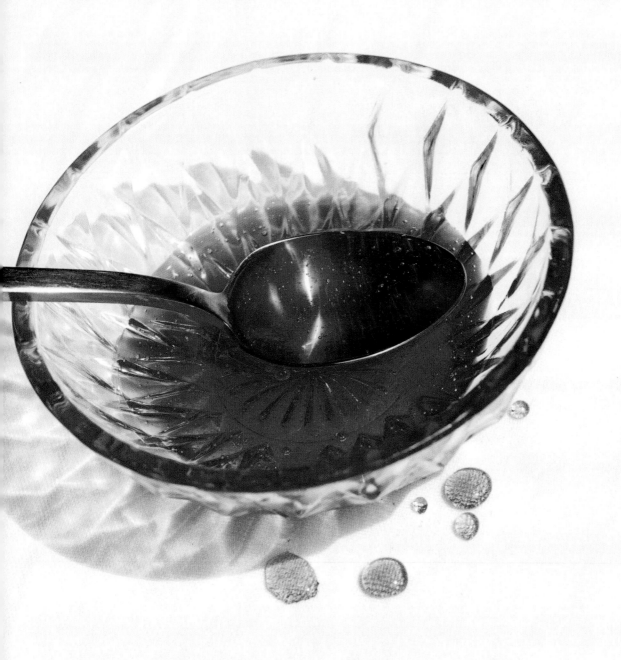
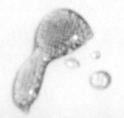

RAW HONEY

Honey

WILL IMPROVE

YOUR CIRCULATION . . .

everywhere

RAW ORGANIC HONEY IS AN ESSENTIAL PART OF ANY HEALING PANTRY.

Unlike the squeeze-honey bear version, raw honey isn't heated to high temperatures or filtered, which preserves its powerful nutrients and enzymes that possess antioxidant and antibiotic properties. Raw honey, which contains all the main essential amino acids, strengthens the immune system, combats allergies, alleviates respiratory problems, aids digestion, provides a gentle energy boost, is a natural remedy for cuts and burns, and keeps the body looking and feeling youthful and strong. Always buy bee-friendly honeys. But if you prefer to avoid honey, you can always swap it out for maple syrup.

CHICKPEA SCRAMBLE

SERVES 4

FOR THE ROASTED VEGETABLES

1 cup (125 g) shiitake
 mushrooms, stems removed
 and caps thinly sliced

2 teaspoons extra-virgin
 olive oil

2 teaspoons tamari soy sauce

Himalayan salt

5 medium stalks asparagus,
 trimmed and cut into
 1-inch (2.5 cm) pieces

½ cup (75 g) cherry tomatoes,
 halved

½ teaspoon store-bought
 harissa paste, or more to
 taste

FOR THE CHICKPEA SCRAMBLE

2 teaspoons extra-virgin
 olive oil

¾ cup (70 g) chickpea flour

1 tablespoon tocotrienols

¼ teaspoon Himalayan salt,
 or more to taste

1½ cups (360 ml) vegetable
 stock

1 tablespoon tamari soy sauce

2 tablespoons minced chives

Microgreens, for garnish

This is a cheeky take on the time-honored breakfast staple, except using protein-filled chickpeas. These little legumes have been part of traditional healing diets for more than seventy-five hundred years, and for good reason—in addition to being full of digestion-aiding fiber and energy-boosting protein, chickpeas have an alkalizing, anti-inflammatory effect on the body that fends off disease. They're also rich in zinc, which is an essential trace mineral that plays a major role in speeding up healing and protecting against free-radical damage. And, for good measure, we whisk in a dose of tocos—short for tocotrienols—a bioavailable source of vitamin E that nourishes the skin and connective tissues while helping to escort toxins out of the body. A breakfast that will surely be able to stand the test of time!

1   Make the vegetables: Preheat the oven to 400°F (205°C). Line a baking sheet with parchment paper and set aside.

2   In a medium bowl, toss the mushrooms with 1 teaspoon of the oil, 1 teaspoon of the tamari, and a pinch of salt. Arrange the mushrooms in a single layer on half of the baking sheet and roast for 15 minutes. While the mushrooms roast, add the asparagus to the same bowl and toss with the remaining 1 teaspoon of oil, the remaining 1 teaspoon of tamari, and a pinch of salt. After the mushrooms have been in the oven for 15 minutes, add the asparagus to the baking sheet and roast until the asparagus is just tender and the mushrooms are nicely browned and beginning to crisp, about 5 more minutes.

RECIPE CONTINUES

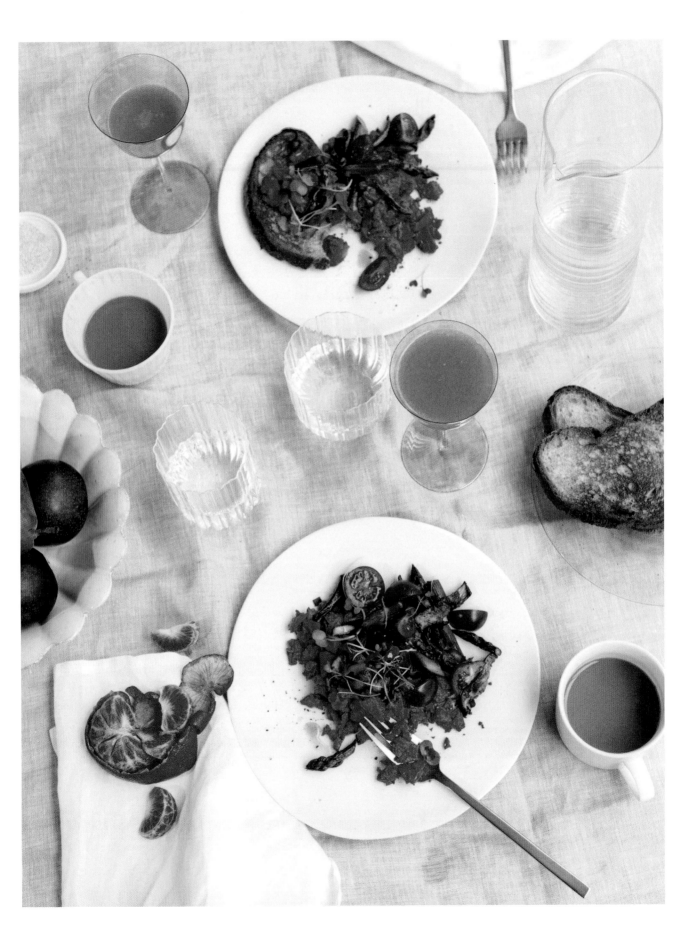

3   In a large bowl, toss together the roasted mushrooms and asparagus with the tomatoes and the harissa. If you want more spice, feel free to add more harissa to your liking. Set aside.

4   Make the chickpea scramble: Coat a baking sheet with 1 teaspoon of the oil and set aside.

5   In a medium pot, combine the flour, tocos, salt, vegetable stock, and tamari over medium-high heat and whisk together. Continue whisking as you bring the mixture to a simmer and the consistency thickens. Switch to a spatula and cook, stirring constantly, for 10 minutes, or until the mixture is thick like a batter and no longer has a raw taste. Fold in the chives and season with additional salt, if desired. Gently spread the mixture over the oiled baking sheet (don't worry if you can't get it completely smooth) and allow to cool. Once cool, crumble the chickpea mixture into pieces—it should resemble scrambled eggs.

6   Divide the scramble among 4 bowls. Top with the vegetable mixture, sprinkle with the microgreens, and serve hot.

SAKARA EVERYTHING BAGELS WITH GARLIC SCHMEAR

Sometimes you just need a bagel. But your love for a bagel generally isn't returned. Especially when topped with highly processed cream cheese, it can wreak havoc on your digestive and immune systems. Now that we're New Yorkers, we had to create a version where the love was mutual: this unprocessed alternative, along with a creamy cashew-garlic spread that gets cheesy, tangy flavor (and essential B vitamins) from nutritional yeast. We love topping ours off with quick-pickled red onions and highly recommend slicing up some watermelon radishes for their spicy kick, super-hydrating properties, and bold pink color, which pretties up everything à la smoked salmon. We're also partial to cucumbers and microgreens to get our green in.

MAKES 10 BAGELS

FOR THE EVERYTHING TOPPING

2 teaspoons gluten-free rolled oats

1 teaspoon white sesame seeds

1 teaspoon poppy seeds

½ teaspoon sunflower seeds

¼ teaspoon Himalayan salt

FOR THE BAGELS

1 packet (1½ teaspoons) dry active yeast

2 tablespoons plus 1 teaspoon coconut palm sugar

3 tablespoons flaxseed meal

1 tablespoon sunflower oil

2 teaspoons apple cider vinegar

Cornmeal, for dusting

¾ cup (90 g) millet flour

¾ cup (70 g) oat flour

⅓ cup (55 g) potato starch

⅓ cup (45 g) arrowroot powder

1 teaspoon baking powder

2½ teaspoons baking soda

½ teaspoon Himalayan salt

FOR THE SCHMEAR

1 cup (120 g) raw cashews, soaked overnight and drained

2 cloves garlic, peeled

1 tablespoon nutritional yeast

Pinch of red pepper flakes

Himalayan salt

FOR THE PICKLED RED ONIONS

½ cup (120 ml) apple cider vinegar

1 tablespoon wildflower honey

1½ teaspoons Himalayan salt

1 small red onion, thinly sliced

FOR FINISHING

Thinly sliced watermelon radish (optional)

Thinly sliced cucumber (optional)

Microgreens (optional)

RECIPE CONTINUES

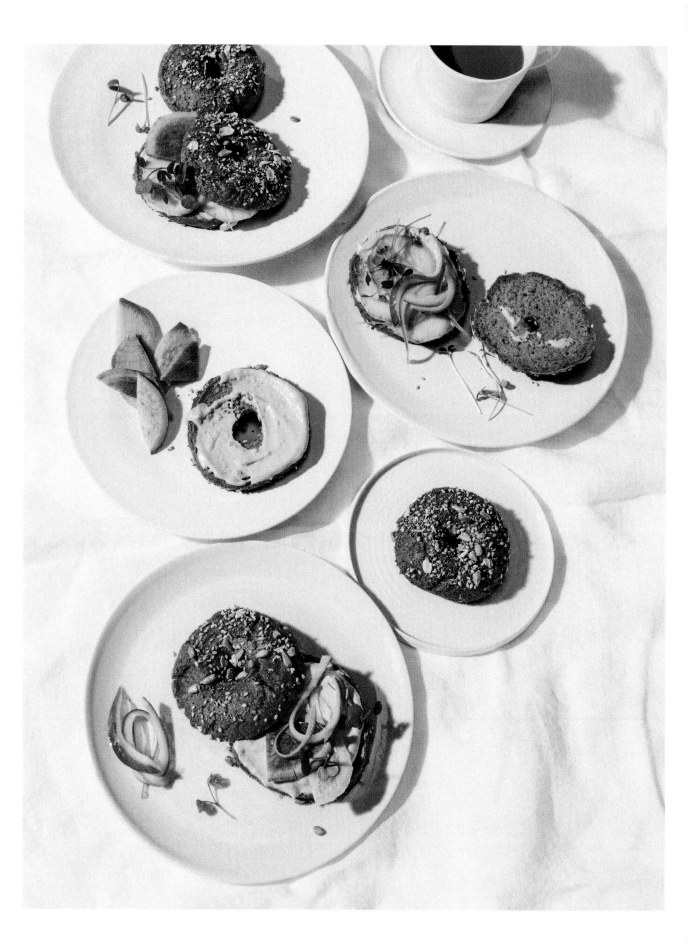

1   Make the everything topping: In a small bowl, combine all the ingredients and set aside.

2   Make the bagels: In a small bowl, combine the yeast and 1 teaspoon of the sugar. Add 1 cup (240 ml) of warm water and allow the mixture to bubble, 10 to 15 minutes. Stir in the flaxseed meal, oil, and vinegar, then allow 5 minutes for the mixture to thicken.

3   Line a baking sheet with parchment paper and lightly dust with cornmeal. Set aside.

4   In a large bowl, whisk together the millet flour, oat flour, potato starch, arrowroot powder, baking powder, ½ teaspoon of the baking soda, and salt. Add the yeast mixture and stir with a spatula until completely combined.

5   Divide the dough into 10 evenly sized balls. Use your thumb to create a hole in the middle of each ball and gently form the dough into a bagel shape. Lay the bagels on the cornmeal-dusted baking sheet and flatten the dough slightly until each bagel is about ½ inch (12 mm) thick. Cover the bagels with a clean towel and allow the dough to rise for 45 minutes.

6   Preheat the oven to 425°F (220°C).

7   Fill a large pot with 8 cups (2 L) of water and bring to a boil. Add the remaining 2 tablespoons of the sugar and the remaining 2 teaspoons of the baking soda. Working in small batches so you don't overcrowd the pot, carefully add the bagels to the boiling water. Boil for 30 seconds on each side, then use a slotted spoon to scoop them out and shake off any excess water. Return them to the parchment-lined baking sheet and immediately sprinkle with the everything topping.

8   Bake the bagels for 20 to 25 minutes, or until golden brown. Allow them to cool completely on a wire rack before storing them at room temperature in an airtight container for up to 3 days, or in the freezer for up to 1 month.

9   Make the schmear: In a blender or food processor, combine the cashews, garlic, nutritional yeast, red pepper flakes, and a pinch of salt with ½ cup (120 ml) of water. Blend until creamy. Adjust the consistency with more water, if necessary, and taste. Add more salt, if desired.

10   Make the pickled red onions: In a medium bowl, whisk together the vinegar, honey, and salt with 1 cup (120 ml) of water until the honey and salt dissolve. Place the onions in a jar and pour the vinegar mix over. Let the onions sit at room temperature for at least 1 hour, or chill them overnight. Any leftovers will last pretty much forever in your fridge.

11   Serve: Slice bagels in half and spread with the schmear. Load them up with your desired toppings, such as the pickled red onions, watermelon radish, cucumber, and microgreens, if using, and enjoy.

SUPERFOOD PANCAKES WITH CHIA-BERRY COMPOTE AND LEMON-CASHEW CRÈME

FOR THE CHIA-BERRY COMPOTE

1 cup (125 g) raspberries

1 cup (200 g) strawberries, hulled

1 tablespoon raw honey

⅓ cup (55 g) chia seeds

FOR THE LEMON-CASHEW CRÈME

1 cup (120 g) raw cashews, soaked overnight and drained

1 tablespoon coconut oil

1 tablespoon maple syrup

1 teaspoon pure vanilla extract

Zest of 1 lemon

FOR THE PANCAKES

¼ cup (35 g) flaxseed meal

1¾ cups (210 g) buckwheat flour or gluten-free flour

3 teaspoons baking powder

¼ teaspoon baking soda

½ cup (120 ml) cashew or almond milk

3 tablespoons coconut oil

When we created Sakara, our intention was to provide nutrition *and* joy. We didn't want anything to be off-limits, especially a quintessential breakfast option like pancakes. In the spirit of balance, we've created the perfect blend of indulgence and sustenance: a piping-hot tall stack loaded with plant-derived protein, with layers of fresh berry and chia compote and creamy, citrus-spiked crème slathered in between, like a breakfast-y naked cake.

1   Make the chia-berry compote: In a food processor, combine the raspberries and strawberries and pulse until chunky. Transfer to a small saucepan over low heat. Add the honey and simmer until the sauce thickens, about 5 minutes. Remove from the heat, stir in the chia seeds, and allow the mixture to cool.

2   Make the lemon-cashew crème: In a food processor, combine all the ingredients and blend until smooth. Set aside.

3   Make the pancakes: Make a flax egg by mixing together the flaxseed meal with 1¼ cups (300 ml) of water. Let the mixture sit until thickened, about 2 minutes.

4   In a large bowl, combine the flour, baking powder, and baking soda and whisk together. Pour in the milk and flax egg and stir until the batter is completely smooth.

RECIPE CONTINUES

EAT CLEAN

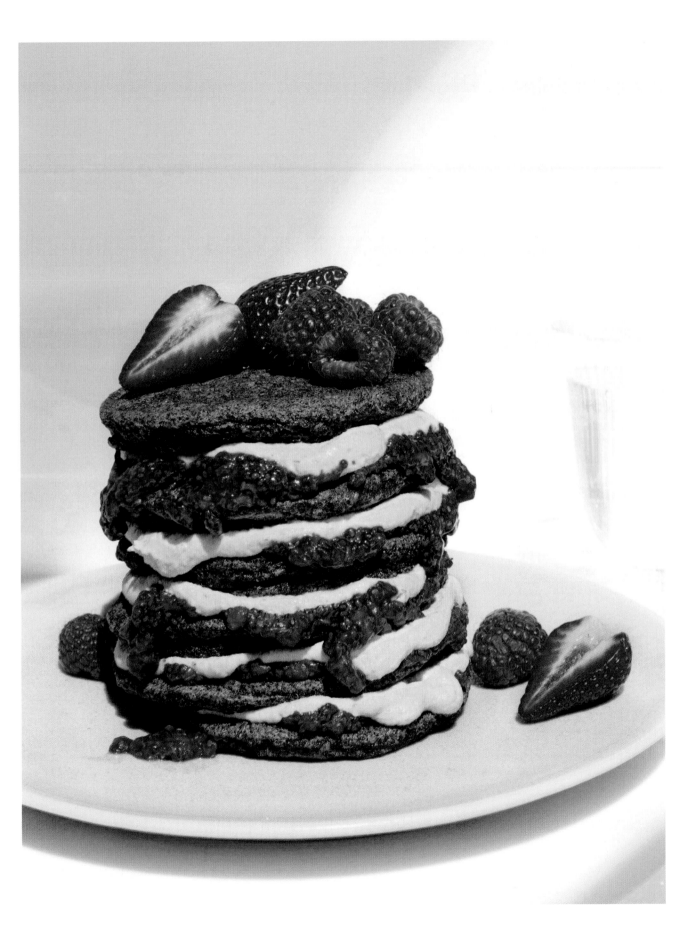

5   In a large skillet, heat 1 tablespoon of the oil over medium-high heat. Drop the batter by the ¼ cup-ful (60 ml) into the pan. About 3 pancakes will fit in the pan at one time. Cook until bubbles form in the batter, about 1 minute. Use a spatula to flip the pancakes and continue cooking until there's no loose batter in the middle, about 2 minutes more. Repeat until the batter is finished, adding more oil to the pan before each new batch.

6   Prepare a piping bag or make your own by snipping a ½-inch-wide (12 mm) opening in the corner of a large Ziploc bag. Fill the bag with the crème. Lay one pancake on a serving plate, spread it with about a tablespoon of the compote, and then pipe the top with the crème. Continue alternating until you've run out of pancakes. Store leftover pancakes and toppings in the fridge for up to 3 days.

CHIA SEEDS

THESE
little beauties
are among the
healthiest foods
on earth

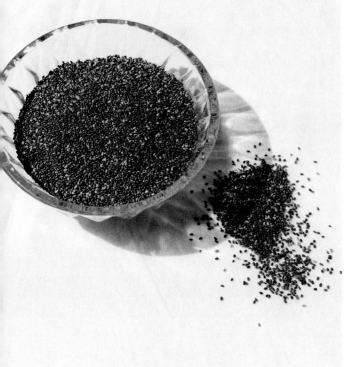

The Aztecs and the Mayans revered them as sacred, using them in almost everything they ate because of their ability to provide sustainable energy. The name *chia* actually comes from the Mayan word for strength.

Just two tablespoons of chia seeds contain an impressive eleven grams of fiber, which means smooth sailing in the digestion department. Because of all that fiber, these seeds can absorb up to twelve times their weight in water and create a sort of gel that expands in your stomach, helping to feed friendly bacteria, aiding in more comfortable digestive and elimination processes, and contributing to hours of post-meal satiation (in other words, they help you feel fuller longer). Then these slippery seeds wind their way through your system, depositing nutrients like myricetin, quercetin, kaempferol, and caffeic acid (all of which are known for their antioxidant, anti-inflammatory, and anti-cancer properties) and flushing out anything your body has no business holding on to.

Chia seeds can stay fresh for up to two years because the antioxidants in their little shells act as natural preservatives for the heavy concentration of fats they contain, which would otherwise go rancid quickly (as is the case with your quickly browning avocados). Store your seeds in the fridge for a prolonged shelf life. Chias are quick and easy to use for any meal. Our favorite way to utilize them is by making overnight chia seed pudding with nut or coconut milk, or tossing a couple of spoonfuls of chias into a smoothie. They're also great sprinkled on top of salads and soups as a way to boost the nutrient density of just about any meal.

BREAKFAST

53

SPICED APPLE-QUINOA MUFFINS WITH COCONUT CRUMBLE

FOR THE CRUMBLE TOPPING

½ cup (45 g) rolled oats

2 tablespoons coconut palm sugar

1 tablespoon coconut oil, melted

1 tablespoon chia seeds

FOR THE MUFFINS

¼ cup (50 g) plus 1 tablespoon flaxseed meal

¾ cup (150 g) red or yellow lentils

1 cup (115 g) almond flour

¾ cup (85 g) quinoa flour

⅓ cup (35 g) raw walnuts

2 teaspoons baking powder

1 teaspoon baking soda

1 teaspoon ground cinnamon

½ teaspoon ground cloves (optional)

¼ teaspoon Himalayan salt

¼ cup (240 ml) unsweetened applesauce

¼ cup (60 ml) almond butter

¾ cup (180 ml) raw honey

¼ cup (60 ml) coconut oil

1¼ cups (150 g) finely chopped apples (we like Braeburn, Granny Smith, and Pink Lady)

These lovely muffins contain two superfood secret weapons: quinoa flour, which stabilizes blood sugar and provides the gut with essential daily fiber, and lentils, which add protein (without any lentil-y flavor). The finishing touch: cinnamon, cloves, and apples. Apples are packed with beautifying phytonutrients, antioxidants, and soluble fiber (the good kind that keeps things moving and grooving through your digestive system). Great for breakfast or for when traveling—if you know what we mean.

1   Make the crumble topping: In a medium bowl, combine all the ingredients. Set aside.

2   Make the muffins: Preheat the oven to 325°F (165°C). Line 12 muffin cups. In a small bowl, whisk together 1 tablespoon of the flaxseed meal with 2½ tablespoons of water. Let the mixture sit for a minute or two to thicken.

3   In a medium saucepan over medium heat, combine the lentils with 2 cups (480 ml) of water. Bring to a boil, reduce to a simmer, and cook until the lentils break down and most of the water is absorbed, 15 to 20 minutes. Mash the lentils with a potato masher until smooth and set aside to cool.

4   In a large bowl, stir together the flours, remaining ¼ cup (35 g) of flaxseed meal, walnuts, baking powder, baking soda, cinnamon, cloves (if using), and salt.

5   In another large bowl, combine the lentil puree with the flaxseed and water mixture, applesauce, almond buter, honey, oil, and chopped apples. Mix well. Stir the dry ingredients into the wet and mix just until all the flour is incorporated and the batter is smooth. Divide the mixture among the muffin cups by the ½ cup-ful (120 ml). Sprinkle the crumble topping over each muffin and bake for 20 minutes, or until the tops are golden and a toothpick inserted into the middle of a muffin comes out clean.

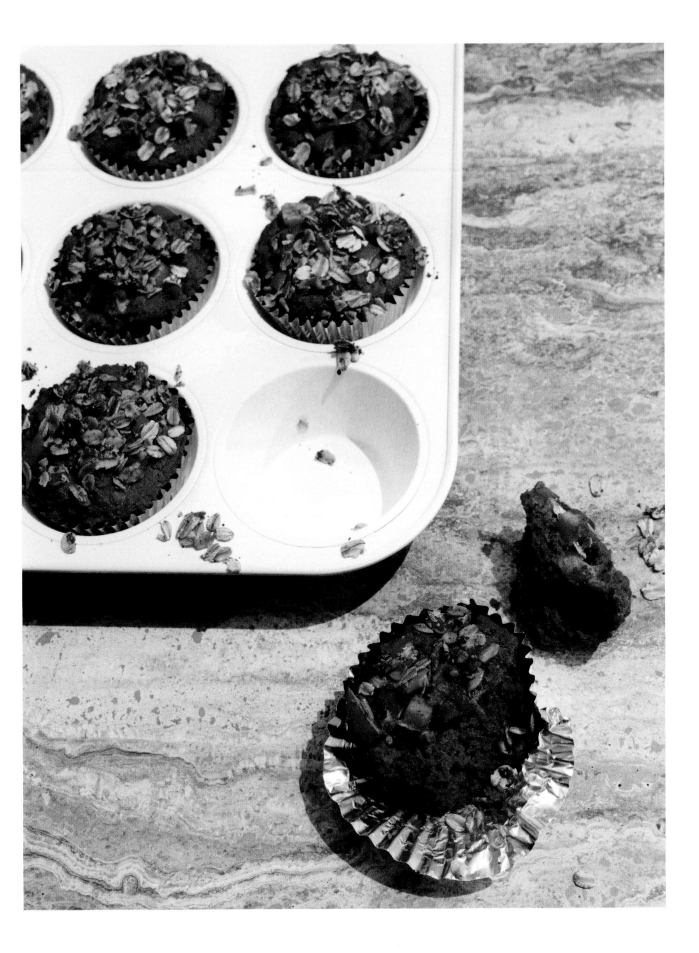

BEAUTY ELIXIR

7 hibiscus tea bags, or
    2 tablespoons plus
     1 teaspoon loose tea

2 tablespoons wildflower honey

1 teaspoon MSM

½ teaspoon camu camu powder

½ teaspoon schisandra berry

1 tablespoon fresh lemon juice

Berries embody the very essence of beauty. They are the precious fruit that emerges from the womb of the flower, delicate and succulent. Even their name—which overlaps with *bare* in etymology—suggests something revealed, sensual, and exultant. This edible flesh from nature's most seductive creations lends us their allure. The schisandra berry has long been prized for its beauty-making prowess, having the ability to nourish the skin from within and reverse the wear and tear on our cells and tissues that can accelerate signs of aging. Camu camu, another superberry, also works to slow the body's clock and tame inflammation. The result? Supple, glowing skin. We've harnessed these berries' power in this daily tonic. We steep these berries in hibiscus tea, another ally from the flower realm whose antioxidative properties further shield the skin, and we add a dose of MSM (methylsulfonylmethane), an organic sulfur-containing compound that occurs naturally in some green vegetables and is necessary for collagen production. This elixir is sure to manifest the sensuality of a fruit and the beauty of a flower.

In a large pot, combine the tea, honey, MSM, camu camu, and schisandra with 5 cups (1.2 L) of water. Bring the mixture to a boil, remove the pot from the heat, and cover. Let the mixture steep for 15 minutes. Strain and stir in the lemon juice. Cool the elixir to room temperature before storing in the fridge for up to 5 days. Enjoy this elixir as you would tea—chilled, warmed, or at room temperature. You can also use it as the base for smoothies, or mix it with a touch of nut milk for a fuller-bodied tonic.

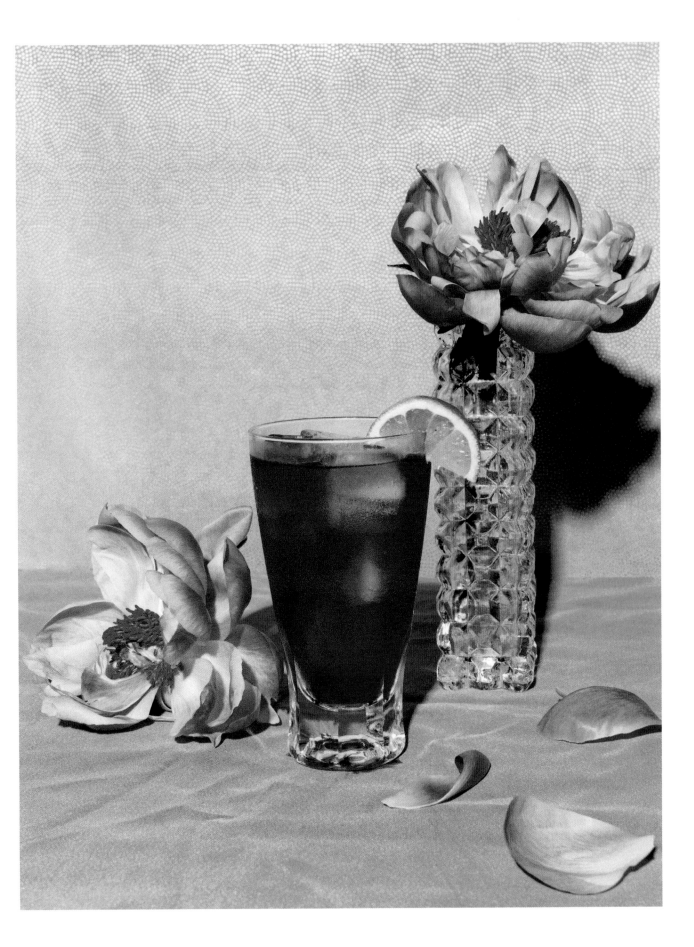

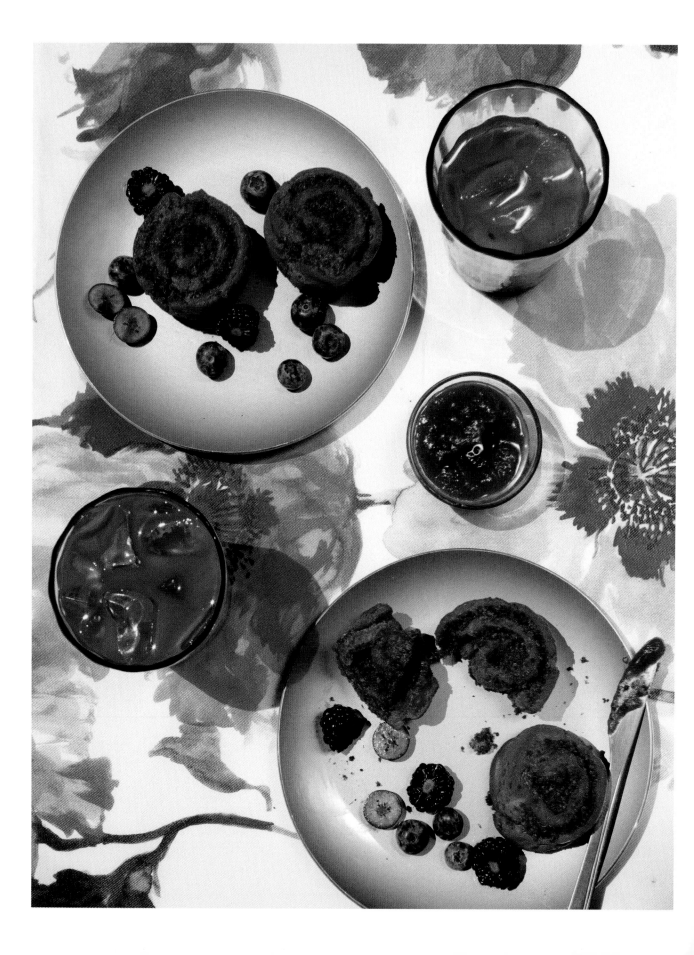

SEXY CINNAMON ROLLS

What makes these cinnamon rolls so sexy? Aside from getting to enjoy a steaming hot, sweet, sticky, cinnamon-spiced bun slathered in date caramel? We spike our version with *Mucuna pruriens*, a powerful seed that has benefits for your brain *and* your libido. It's been used for centuries in Ayurveda, Chinese traditional medicine, and shamanic medicine due to its potent stores of L-dopa, an amino acid and hormone that helps the brain create more feel-good transmitters while stoking the sensual fire. When you make a batch of these rolls, we challenge you to get in touch with your sexual energy and harness it to power your day. Wear your naughtiest underwear beneath your suit; spritz on your date-night perfume during the day; send your partner a wicked little text—anything to reignite your stores of fiery, passionate, powerfully creative energy.

MAKES 6 ROLLS

FOR THE DOUGH

¼ cup (60 ml) plus
2 tablespoons almond milk

1 packet (2¼ teaspoons) dry active yeast

2 tablespoons plus 1 teaspoon coconut oil, melted, plus more for the pan

2 tablespoons coconut palm sugar

⅓ cup (55 g) potato starch

⅓ cup (30 g) oat flour

2 tablespoons white rice flour

2 tablespoons tapioca starch, plus more for dusting

1½ teaspoons baking powder

1 teaspoon *Mucuna pruriens*

¼ teaspoon baking soda

¼ teaspoon xanthan gum

¼ teaspoon Himalayan salt

2 tablespoons unsweetened applesauce

¼ teaspoon pure vanilla extract

FOR THE FILLING

¼ cup (50 g) coconut palm sugar

2 tablespoons coconut oil

⅓ cup (30 g) psyllium husk powder

1½ teaspoons ground cinnamon

¼ teaspoon almond milk, if needed

FOR THE CARAMEL

1 cup (175 g) pitted dates, soaked in boiling water for 20 minutes and drained

½ tablespoon maple syrup

½ teaspoon Himalayan salt

RECIPE CONTINUES

59

1   Make the dough: In a small pot, gently warm the milk over medium-low heat until it is warm to the touch. Remove from heat and add the yeast plus ½ tablespoon of the oil and ½ tablespoon of the sugar. Set aside to proof for 10 minutes, until the yeast is frothy. Add 1½ tablespoons of the oil and the remaining 1½ tablespoons of sugar.

2   In the bowl of a stand mixer fitted with the paddle attachment, combine the potato starch, oat flour, rice flour, tapioca starch, baking powder, *Mucuna pruriens*, baking soda, xanthan gum, and salt. Mix on low speed for about 30 seconds to evenly combine.

3   Add the yeast mixture, applesauce, and vanilla to the bowl and mix on high speed for 5 to 6 minutes. The dough will be pretty tacky. Cover the bowl with plastic wrap and refrigerate overnight.

4   Make the filling: In a medium bowl, blend together the sugar and oil until smooth. Stir in the psyllium husk powder and cinnamon. Add the milk, if needed, to adjust the consistency—you're looking for a crumbly mixture that sticks to itself slightly.

5   Assemble and bake the rolls: Cover a clean work surface with plastic wrap and sprinkle with tapioca starch. Turn out the dough onto the plastic and cover with a second sheet of plastic wrap. Using a rolling pin or your hands, shape the dough into a roughly 8 by 9-inch (20 by 23 cm) rectangle, about ⅛ inch (3 mm) thick. Remove the top sheet of plastic wrap and gently spread the dough with the remaining 1 teaspoon of the oil. Scatter the filling evenly and generously over the top of the dough. You may not use all the filling, and that's okay. Using the plastic wrap to help lift one of the short ends of the dough, tightly roll the dough into a cylinder. Leave the roll wrapped in plastic and transfer it to the refrigerator to chill for 30 minutes.

6   Make the caramel: In a blender, combine the dates, maple syrup, and salt with ½ cup (120 ml) of warm water and blend until smooth.

7   Preheat the oven to 325°F (165°C). Grease 6 tins of a muffin pan with oil.

8   Slice the dough into six 1½-inch (4 cm) pieces. Carefully place the rolls swirl side up in each of the muffin cups. It's okay if the dough tears—simply pinch it back together in the pan. Bake for 35 minutes, or until the tops are golden and slightly firm to the touch.

9   Drizzle or slather the rolls with the caramel while still warm. Enjoy steaming hot.

COCONUT

Coconut is one of THE MOST *multitalented* *healers* *in the* *plant world*

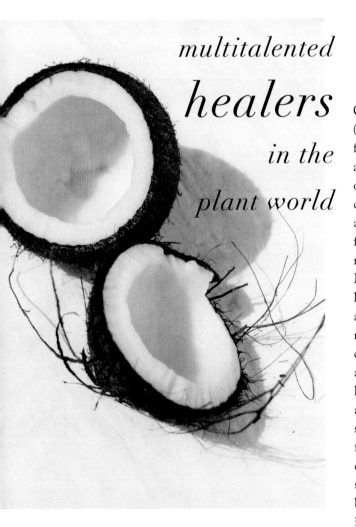

COCONUT OIL, COCONUT BUTTER, AND DRIED COCONUT HAVE ANTIBACTERIAL AND IMMUNE-STRENGTHENING PROPERTIES.

Coconut oil contains lauric acid and MCTs (or medium-chain triglycerides, aka healthy fats that can function as anti-inflammatory agents), which fight yeasts, parasites, bacterial overgrowth, and even common viruses like the cold. Coconut is hydrating and rich in fiber and nutrients, and especially magical in its raw, fresh form. Young coconut meat is high in vitamins, amino acids, and antioxidants—along with MCTs—plus it helps the body boost its levels of healthy cholesterol. That's right—the body actually needs cholesterol in order to maintain optimal hormonal balance, but not all cholesterol is created equal. Coconut's healthy fats and amino acids supercharge your neurotransmitters, which helps boost and stabilize your moods, fend off anxiety and depression, minimize the damage of stress, and prevent memory loss. These healthy fats lend a hand to your liver too, taking its detoxifying powers to the next level while also strengthening overall digestive health. Another bonus of cracking into a fresh young coconut is the coconut water. Super-hydrating coconut water is packed with electrolytes, which are important for the optimal health of our cardiovascular, nervous, and immune systems, as well as for maintaining overall balance in the body—not to mention that it's an incredible cure for a hangover. (Hey, it happens. Just make sure you have a coconut handy!)

ORGASMIC COCONUT YOGURT

2 cups (200 g) fresh young Thai coconut meat

½ cup (120 ml) coconut water

1 tablespoon fresh lime juice

Pinch of Himalayan or fine-grain salt

½ teaspoon probiotic powder (about 3 capsules, optional)

Coconut nectar, honey, or maple syrup (optional)

The name really says it all! This yogurt is lusciously smooth, creamy, and tangy thanks to coconut's healthy fat content and natural probiotic activation. Serve it chilled under a sprinkling of granola, spooned over fresh fruit, or drizzled into soups—or lick it straight from the spoon. As everyone at Sakara can attest, you should be prepared to fall in love.

Be sure to use young coconut meat to get the creamy, orgasmic texture we're talking about.

1   In a blender, combine the coconut meat, coconut water, lime juice, and salt and puree until smooth. At this point, you can enjoy the yogurt and store it in the fridge for up to a week. If you want to culture the yogurt, transfer it to a jar or bowl. Empty the probiotic capsules into the yogurt and use a wooden or plastic spoon to stir until the powder is completely incorporated. (A metal spoon can dull the lively spark of your probiotics.)

2   Cover the mixture with cheesecloth or a clean kitchen towel and leave the yogurt at room temperature to culture for at least 24 hours or up to 48 hours. The longer it rests, the thicker and tangier your yogurt will get. If your house is cooler than 75°F (24°C), you can leave the yogurt in your oven with just the oven light on.

3   Sample the yogurt occasionally to see if it's tangy to your liking. Once it's satisfactorily cultured, you can sweeten or flavor the yogurt any way you like. We like a small spoonful of coconut nectar, honey, or maple syrup. Cover and store the yogurt in the fridge, where it will continue to thicken, for up to 1 week.

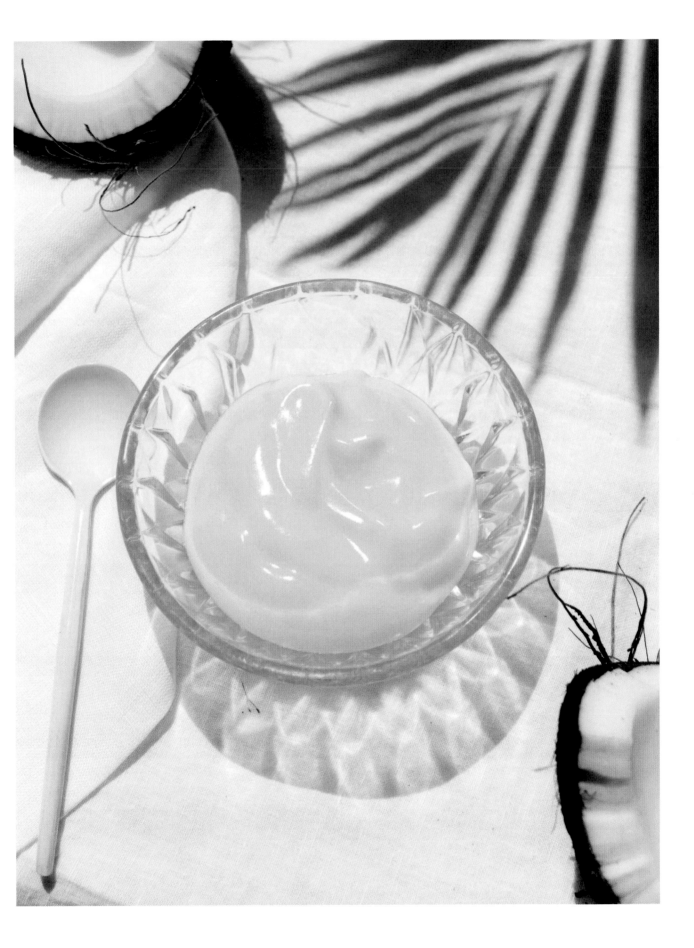

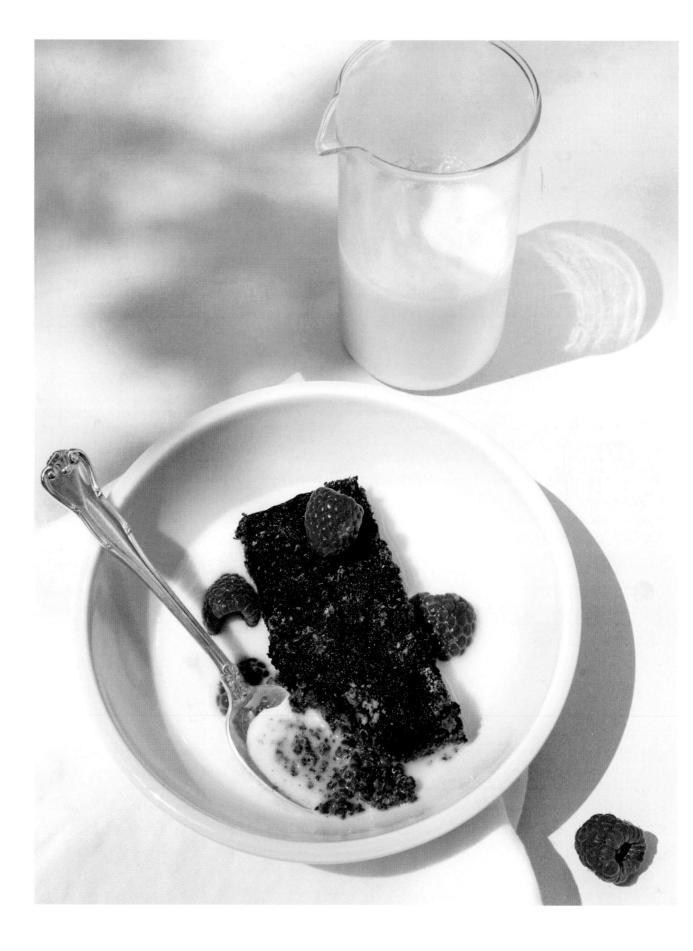

DANIELLE'S COCOA-QUINOA CAKE SQUARES

1 cup (170 g) uncooked quinoa, or 3 cups (555 g) cooked

1½ cups (360 ml) unsweetened hemp, soy, or nut milk

1 cup (175 g) pitted dates

½ cup (80 g) hulled hemp seeds

½ cup (120 ml) unsweetened applesauce

⅓ cup (30 g) unsweetened cocoa powder

¾ cup (85 g) almond meal or flour

¼ teaspoon Himalayan or fine salt

Fresh raspberries, for serving

Almond milk, for serving

Inspired by Danielle and her husband's intense love for all things cocoa, we came up with a way to have your chocolate breakfast cake and eat it too. These bars are as rich and full-bodied as your favorite patisserie treat yet harness the protein power of quinoa and the gentle sweetness of dates. They also include almonds, which are packed with magnesium to gently wake you up and keep you cool, calm, and collected all day long, not to mention provide skin-beautifying vitamin E and healthy fats, plus protein and digestion-friendly fiber.

1   Rinse the uncooked quinoa in a fine-mesh sieve for 1 minute. Transfer to a medium pot, add 2 cups (480 ml) of water, and bring to a boil. Reduce the heat to medium-low and cover, simmering, until the water is absorbed, 15 to 20 minutes. Remove the pot from the heat and wait 5 minutes before uncovering the quinoa and fluffing it with a fork.

2   Preheat the oven to 350°F (175°C). Line the bottom of an 8-inch-square (20 cm) baking pan with parchment paper and set aside.

3   In a blender, combine the milk, dates, hemp seeds, applesauce, cocoa, ½ cup (60 g) of the almond meal, and salt. Blend until smooth. Transfer the mixture to a large bowl and stir in the cooked quinoa.

4   Pour the batter evenly into the prepared pan and sprinkle the remaining ¼ cup (25 g) of almond meal over the top. Bake until the cake is firmly set, about 1 hour. Let the cake cool slightly before using the parchment to lift it out. Let the cake cool completely on a metal cooling rack, about 1 hour. Slice into 1 by 2-inch (2.5 by 5 cm) bars. Serve with raspberries and almond milk. Store any leftovers in an airtight container in the fridge for up to 5 days. Enjoy alone or warm in a bowl with cold almond milk and a spoon.

WHITNEY'S GREEN BARS

MAKES 6 BARS

½ cup (65 g) raw pumpkin seeds

½ cup (70 g) raw sunflower seeds

1 ripe banana

2 dates, pitted

½ cup (45 g) unsweetened shredded coconut

½ teaspoon chlorella

¼ teaspoon Himalayan salt

Our version of a grain-free granola bar features energy-sustaining pumpkin and sunflower seeds, naturally sweet banana and shredded coconut, and one of our favorite secret weapons: chlorella. This vibrant green algae is one of the most nutrient-dense foods on the planet thanks to its concentration of protein, amino acids, iron, vitamin A, and zinc. But it's the supercharged chlorophyll in the chlorella that makes it so special. It's not only what gives these bars their deep green color, it's a magical plant pigment that captures the sun's energy and turns it into usable nourishment (aka photosynthesis). As amazing as the human body is, that's not something we can do on our own. So when we eat chlorophyll-rich plants (especially leafy greens) or foods with a dose of chlorella (like these bars!), we get to borrow this superpower and find life in the light, straight from the truest source of energy: the sun!

1   Line a baking sheet with parchment paper and set aside.

2   In a food processor, combine the pumpkin and sunflower seeds and pulse until they form a coarse meal. Transfer the mixture to a medium bowl. Add the banana and dates to the food processor (no need to clean it out first) and pulse until just about smooth. With the banana-date mixture still in the food processor, add the seed mixture, coconut, chlorella, and salt and pulse a few times to combine.

3   Using clean hands, form the mixture into 1½ by 4-inch (4 by 10 cm) bars, about ½ inch (12 mm) thick. Transfer the bars to the freezer for 15 minutes, or until firm. Store the bars in the fridge for up to 1 week.

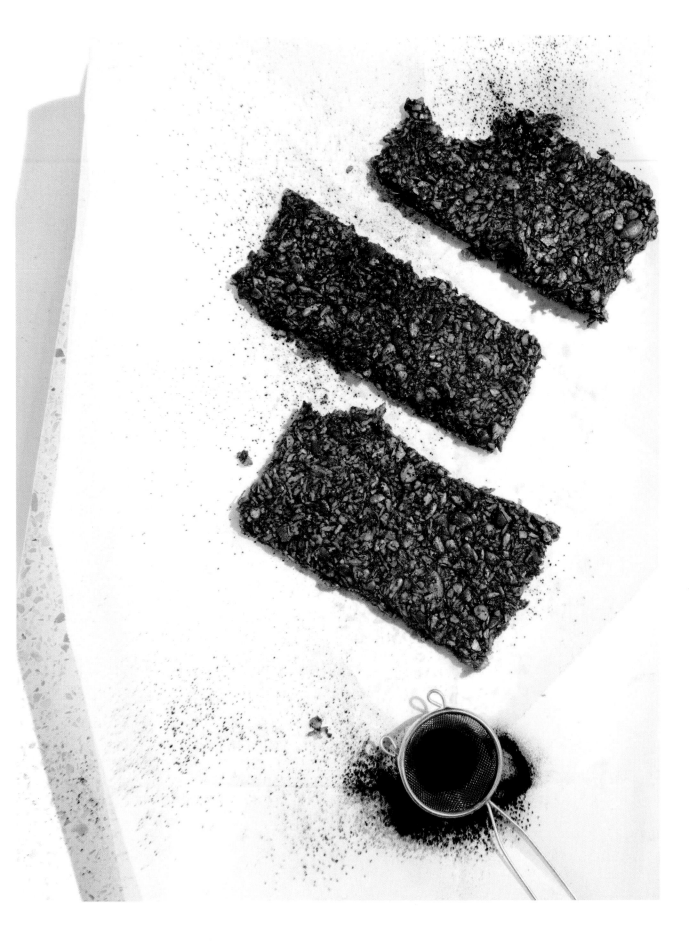

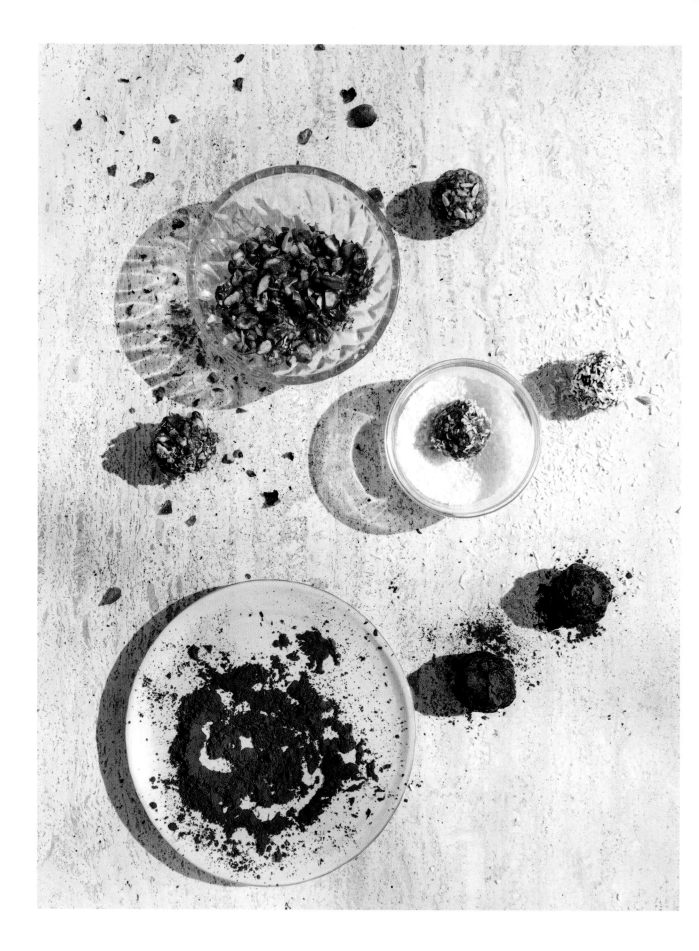

NO-BAKE SUNFLOWER BLISS BITES

MAKES 33 BALLS

2 cups (350 g) pitted dates

1 (16-ounce/470 ml) jar
unsalted, unsweetened
sunflower seed butter

½ teaspoon Himalayan salt

2 cups (180 g) quick-cooking
rolled oats

½ cup (50 g) raw cacao powder
(optional)

½ cup (45 g) unsweetened
shredded coconut
(optional)

½ cup (50 g) shelled, unsalted
pistachios (optional)

Sprinkle of edible dried rose
petals (optional)

These little energy bites were made for a morning in motion. Luckily, you can stash a batch in the fridge or freezer for those moments when time is not a luxury and you, or your little ones, are in need of a sustaining yet delicious (and easy to eat) breakfast. Add a sprinkle of crushed pistachios and dried rose petals, raw cacao powder, or shredded coconut for an extra dose of healthy fats, omega-3s, and protein. Simply blitz, mix, roll, chill, enjoy. Bliss.

1   In a food processor, pulse the dates to finely chop them. You may need to add a few tablespoons of boiling hot water to encourage them. Add the sunflower seed butter and salt and process until smooth.

2   Transfer the mixture to a large bowl and add the oats 1 cup (90 g) at a time, mixing well after each addition. Roll the batter into 1-inch (2.5 cm) balls. If coating the balls with a topping, sprinkle the toppings over individual plates. Roll the balls in the toppings and arrange them on a tray or in a lidded container. Chill them in the refrigerator for at least 30 minutes before enjoying. Store them in the fridge for up to 1 week, or in the freezer for up to 1 month.

BAKED APPLES WITH CINNAMON-OAT CRUMBLE

SERVES 4

½ cup (120 ml) plus 3 tablespoons coconut oil

¼ cup (50 g) coconut palm sugar

½ teaspoon ground cinnamon

½ teaspoon Himalayan salt

¼ cup (30 g) unsalted pistachios, chopped

¼ cup (30 g) slivered almonds

¾ cup (70 g) rolled oats

1 cup (240 ml) fresh-pressed or no-sugar-added apple juice

½ teaspoon pure vanilla extract

Zest of 1 lemon

4 apples (we love Granny Smith, Honeycrisp, or Pink Lady)

Whitney grew up with an apple tree in her yard, and one of her fondest memories is biting into the sweet fruit fresh from the tree. But the ultimate treat was an apple that had been cooked slowly and gently until its flesh softened and its sugars deepened—not unlike the inside of a fresh-baked pie. It's hard to improve on nature's perfection, but to our apples we've added a breakfast-friendly oatmeal-cinnamon crumble with pistachios and almonds.

1   In a food processor, combine ½ cup (120 ml) of the oil with the sugar, cinnamon, and salt. Pulse until the mixture is smooth. Add the nuts and oats and process until a coarse meal forms.

2   In a small saucepan, melt the remaining 3 tablespoons of oil over low heat. Add the apple juice, vanilla, and lemon zest. Simmer for 5 minutes to meld the flavors. Remove from the heat and let the mixture cool slightly.

3   Preheat the oven to 350°F (175°C).

4   Core the apples. We like using a melon baller or spoon to scoop out a slightly larger pocket in the center of the apple so we can squeeze in more filling, but that's optional. Arrange the apples in an ovenproof dish. Divide the stuffing among the apples, packing it tightly in the apples and mounding it over the tops. Pour the apple juice mixture over the apples.

5   Bake for 40 to 50 minutes, or until the apples' flesh is tender, regularly basting them with the cooking juice. Allow to cool slightly before serving.

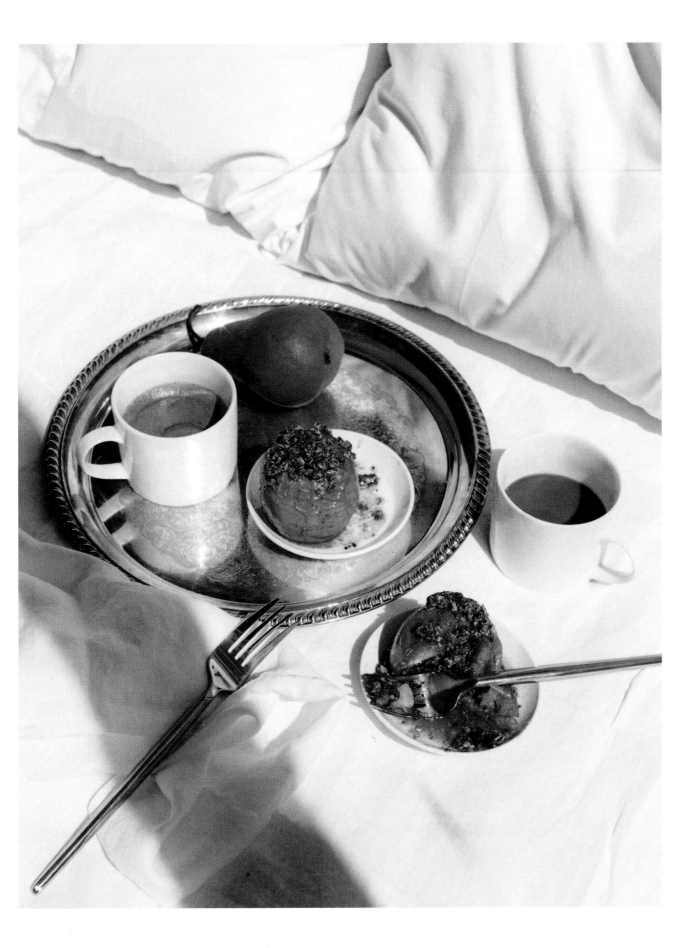

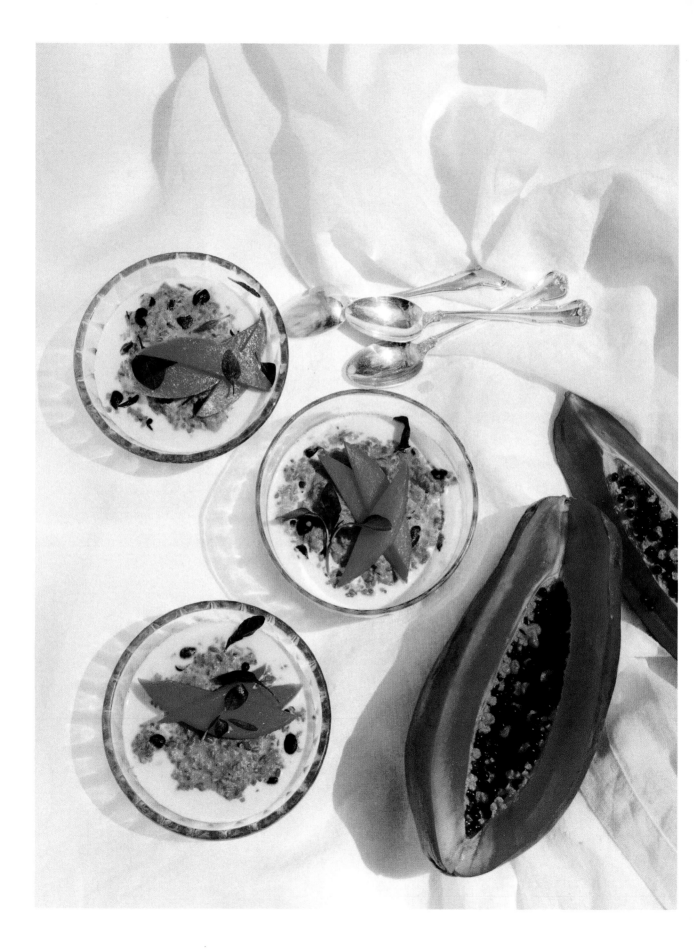

SWEET THAI OATMEAL

1 medium banana

1 cup (90 g) steel-cut gluten-
    free oats

¾ cup (130 g) cooked or
    canned black beans, rinsed
    and drained

2½ cups (540 ml) Thai
    Coconut Mylk (below) or
    unsweetened nut milk

1 teaspoon coconut palm sugar

Pinch of Himalayan salt

1 mango, sliced, for garnish

1 handful microgreens, for
    garnish

This is one of the most delicious recipes ever to be on the Sakara menu, transporting all who indulge by the spoonful to exotic Thai beaches. It calls upon steel-cut oats for a healthy dose of fiber, along with black beans for a traditional Southeast Asian twist and a dose of plant protein to power you through the morning. We simmer the whole lot in coconut milk that's perfumed with the leaves of tropical plants like Thai lime and pandan (which, in addition to imparting sweet flavor, is a natural pain reliever), then top it off with a few slices of fresh mango to inspire daydreams of sun-soaked destinations.

1   In a large pot, mash the banana with a fork until only slightly chunky. Add the oats, beans, milk, sugar, and salt. Stir to combine and bring to a simmer over medium-low heat; reduce the heat to low and cover. Cook, stirring occasionally, until the oats are tender but chewy and about half of the milk has been absorbed, about 20 minutes.

2   Allow the oatmeal to cool slightly before serving with the mango and microgreens.

BREAKFAST

THAI COCONUT MYLK MAKES 4 CUPS (960 ML)

2 (13½-ounce/400 ml) cans
    coconut milk

½ cup (3 g) dried pandan leaves

¼ cup (2 g) dried Thai lime
    leaves

1 tablespoon wildflower honey

Pinch of Himalayan salt

In a medium saucepan, whisk together the milk, pandan leaves, Thai lime leaves, honey, and salt with 1 cup (240 ml) water over medium heat and bring to a rapid simmer. Turn off the heat, cover, and let the mixture steep for 20 minutes. Strain the milk, discarding the leaves. Let the milk cool completely before storing in the fridge for up to 5 days.

FRUIT PARFAIT WITH BEE POLLEN CRUNCH

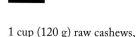

1 cup (120 g) raw cashews, soaked for at least 30 minutes and drained

1 teaspoon wildflower honey

2 tablespoons bee pollen

2 tablespoons goji berries

2 tablespoons unsweetened coconut flakes

½ small pineapple, sliced

1 plum, sliced

1 nectarine, sliced

Juice of ½ lemon

Bees are incredible animals: Buzzing from flower to flower in search of nectar, they coat themselves in pollen and sprinkle the dust over budding blossoms to fertilize and nourish new plants. In this breakfast, you're partaking in the fruits of their labor and reaping the nourishing benefits. Bee pollen is a collection of tiny pellets that worker bees have packed into a lacto-fermented, enzymatically activated food called bee bread. This medicinal substance is stored in hives to sustain young bees but has also been enjoyed by humans because of its natural healing properties and honey-sweet flavor. Bee pollen is usually prescribed to help increase energy and endurance, address a vitamin deficiency (especially during pregnancy), alleviate allergies and asthma, relieve anemia, and improve overall immunity.

We also really love how joyful it is to sprinkle bee pollen over the top of this breakfast sundae, made with a medley of fresh fruit and layers of a honey-flavored cashew whip. The next time you see a bee, bow in gratitude!

1   In a food processor, combine the cashews and honey with ¼ cup (60 ml) of water and process until a smooth cream forms. Set aside.

2   In a small bowl, combine the pollen, berries, and coconut flakes. Set aside.

3   In a medium bowl, toss the sliced pineapple, plum, and nectarine in the lemon juice.

4   Put about a tablespoon of cream in the bottom of 4 parfait glasses or glass bowls. Layer with ½ cup (110 g) of the fruit, another tablespoon of cream, and another ½ cup (110 g) of fruit on top. Sprinkle with the pollen mixture and serve.

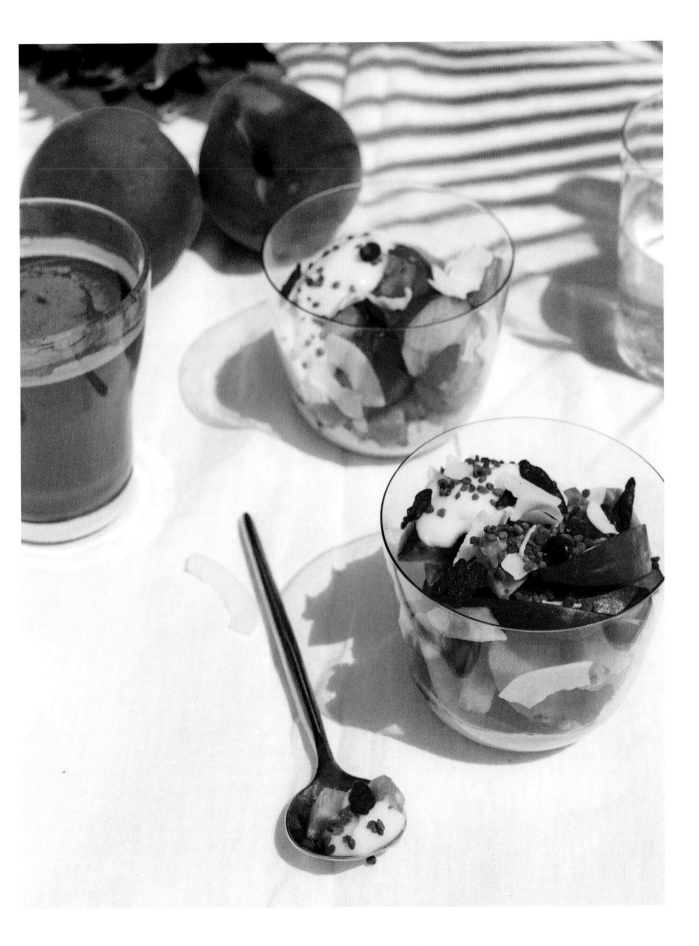

SUPERSEED MUESLI

SERVES 3

2 tablespoons coconut oil

2 tablespoons wildflower honey

1 tablespoon hemp seeds

½ cup (45 g) gluten-free rolled oats

½ cup (60 g) quinoa flakes

¼ cup (35 g) sunflower seeds

1 tablespoon chia seeds

1 tablespoon flaxseeds

1 tablespoon pumpkin seeds

1 tablespoon poppy seeds

1 tablespoon black sesame seeds

½ teaspoon sea buckthorn powder

½ teaspoon vanilla powder or 1 teaspoon pure vanilla extract

½ teaspoon Himalayan salt

½ cup (45 g) dried apples

1 tablespoon dried blackberries or goji berries

Blue Lavender Mylk (page 78), Orgasmic Coconut Yogurt (page 62), or nut milk, for serving

Muesli got its start in the early twentieth century thanks to a Swiss physician looking for an über-healthy breakfast for his patients. For our superseed Sakara version, we updated the classic with quinoa flakes, which deliver tons of plant protein and satisfying fiber; pumpkin seeds for a big dose of magnesium, a mineral required for more than three hundred biochemical reactions in the body; dried blackberries, which on top of providing their anthocyanin antioxidants are such a special treat in this dish; and last but not least, sea buckthorn. Sea buckthorn is extracted from the berries and seeds of the sea buckthorn plant and is powerfully nourishing to the skin as well as to the adrenal system. Thanks to its large natural stores of omega-7s, sea buckthorn is particularly beneficial if you're feeling run-down or depleted. On our Sakara menu, we like to pair this muesli with our infused Blue Lavender Mylk for a delicious and surely "doctor-approved" way to start the day.

1   Preheat the oven to 325°F (165°C). Line a rimmed baking sheet with parchment paper and set aside.

2   In a small pot over low heat, melt together the coconut oil and honey. Set aside.

3   In a large bowl, mix together all the remaining ingredients besides the dried fruit. Stir in the coconut oil and honey mixture until it evenly coats the muesli mixture. Spread the muesli over the prepared baking sheet and bake until golden brown, 15 to 20 minutes, turning the pan halfway through. Let the mixture cool and toss with the dried fruit. Serve with Blue Lavender Mylk, Orgasmic Coconut Yogurt, or nut milk of your choice. The muesli can be stored in an airtight container at room temperature for up to 5 days.

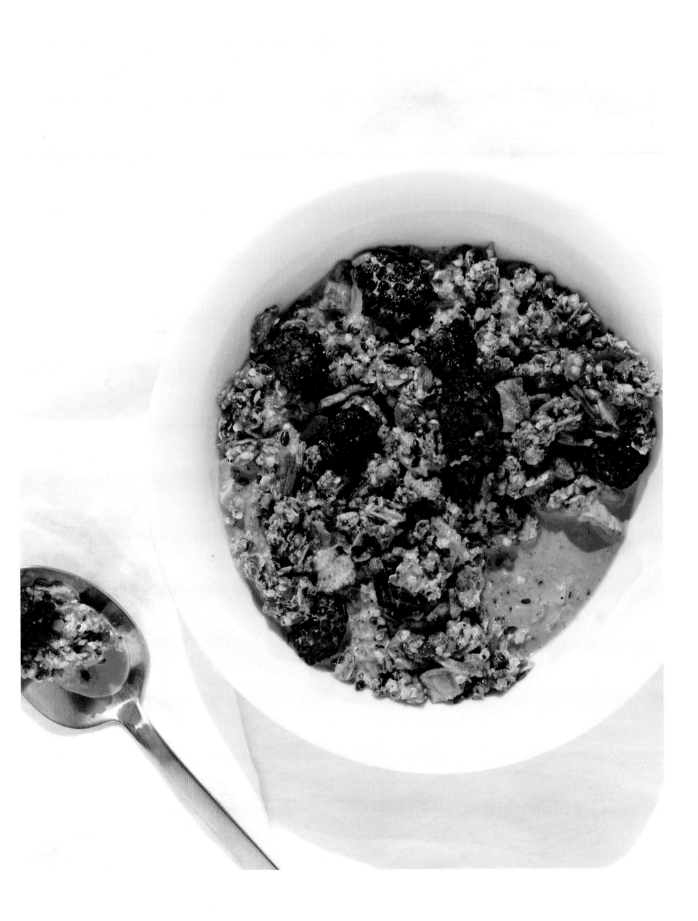

BLUE LAVENDER MYLK

SERVES 3

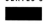

3 cups (720 ml) unsweetened nut milk

1 tablespoon plus 2 teaspoons blue-green algae powder, or substitute for spirulina if you don't have blue-green algae on hand

1 teaspoon dried lavender

2 tablespoons wildflower honey

Don't be alarmed—the bright blue color of this rich almond mylk is totally natural. It comes from blue-green algae, a blue spirulina extract that's packed with body-loving nutrition (and a little bit of magic). It's a rich source of the antioxidant phycocyanin, which lowers inflammation, supports joint health, and rids the body of toxins. We've also added a dash of soothing lavender to this mylk for a beautifully sophisticated flavor, and to ensure you feel at peace with whatever comes your way today.

1   In a medium bowl, whisk together ¾ cup (180 ml) of the milk with the blue-green algae powder. Set aside.

2   Bundle the lavender in a cheesecloth sachet or reusable tea bag.

3   In a small pot, combine the remaining 2¼ cups (540 ml) of milk with the honey and the lavender sachet. Bring the mylk to a gentle simmer over medium-low heat. Remove the pot from the heat and allow the mylk to cool to room temperature. Remove the lavender sachet and stir in the blue-green algae powder mixture until well combined. Store the mylk in the fridge for up to 5 days.

BLUE-GREEN ALGAE

Nourish and *replenish* EVERY ORGAN *in your body*

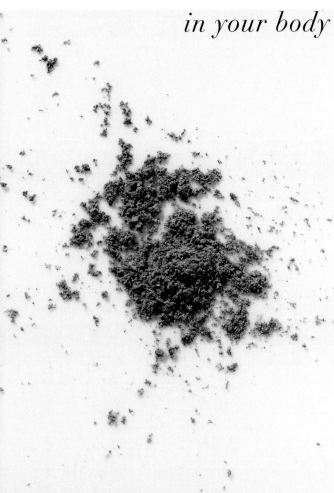

AN INGREDIENT THAT IS PURE MAGIC.

Algae is not only Mother Earth's very first protein source, but it's also the most ancient food on the planet. Algae was the first organism to make use of the sun's energy to photosynthesize food for itself and, consequently, us. Astronauts have been enjoying blue-green algae for more than fifty years because just one gram has the nutritional equivalent of one thousand grams of fruits and veggies, and the United Nations has declared algae to be *the* solution to the world's food shortage because of its rich stores of vitamins, amino acids, and trace minerals. Including just a teaspoon or two in your care regimen immediately nourishes and replenishes every organ in your body, encourages healthy cell turnover, escorts toxins from the body, fights inflammation, delivers a steady stream of energy, and boosts the immune system without overstimulating it. And due to its potent concentration of omega-3s and 6s, blue-green algae helps balance hormones, creating an increased sense of mental clarity and enhanced mood. It also contains a molecule called phenylethylamine (PEA), which contributes to feelings of pleasure. To get the bright robin's-egg blue color in our Blue Lavender Mylk, opt for a blue algae like E3Live's Blue Majik. It is perfect for Instagram photos and tastes great with granola or muesli, blended into tonics, or sipped as is. Enjoy and experience the majik within.

BREAKFAST

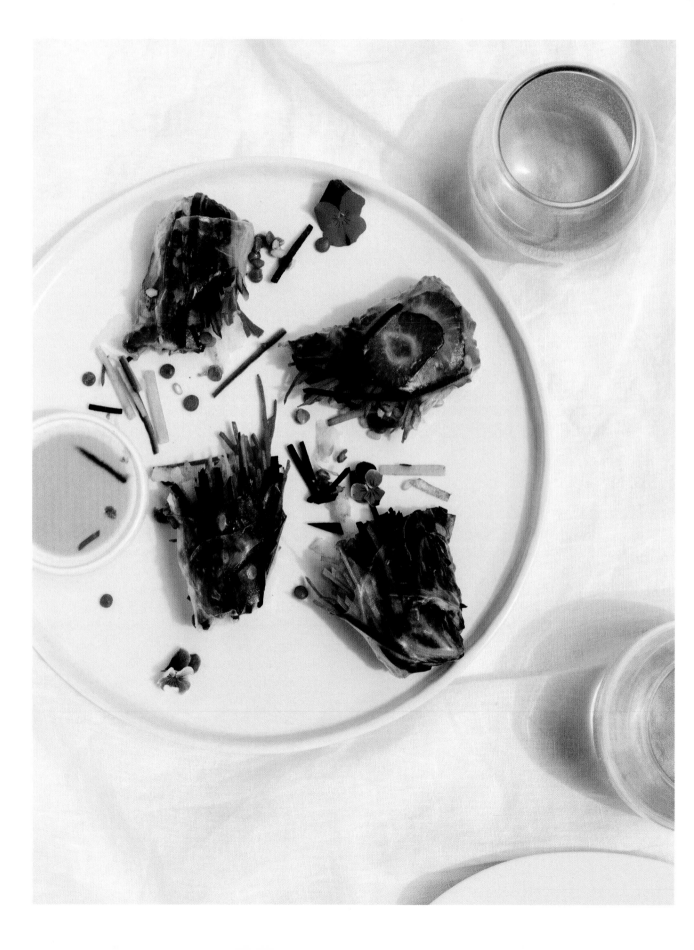

Lunch Sakara lunches are designed to deliver a ton of nutrients to your body—like a daily multivitamin but in the form of a meal. They're also designed to taste good cold or at room temperature, in case you need to eat them at work or on the go!

RAINBOW WRAP, *following page*

RAINBOW WRAP

SERVES 4

FOR THE VINAIGRETTE

1½ tablespoons ume plum vinegar

2½ tablespoons brown rice vinegar

⅓ cup (15 g) roughly chopped fresh ginger

¼ cup (60 ml) plus 1 tablespoon fresh lime juice

1½ tablespoons tamari soy sauce or Bragg Liquid Aminos

½ cup (120 ml) extra-virgin olive oil

2 tablespoons plus 1 teaspoon toasted sesame oil

FOR THE WRAPS

¼ cup (55 g) brown rice

¼ cup (60 ml) plus 2 tablespoons toasted sesame oil

¼ cup (50 g) green lentils

4 (10-inch/25 cm) rice paper wrappers (plus a couple of extras, in case one tears)

½ cup (25 g) chopped fresh cilantro

1 avocado, pitted and sliced

1 cup (150 g) grated red beets

1 cup (150 g) grated carrots

1 cup (150 g) grated daikon

½ cup sliced strawberries

Filled with cooling, hydrating veggies like beets, carrots, and daikon (a spicy winter radish), this spring roll–inspired wrap is not only the perfect light lunch that delivers energy-igniting sustenance; it's helping your body boost its metabolism and optimize digestion too. This wrap also features sesame oil, which has been used for centuries as an antiaging remedy. We recommend enjoying this with Daily Greens (page 33), especially some baby kale tossed with quenching powerhouses cucumber and strawberries, for a meal that leaves you feeling as vibrant and ascendant as a sun shower-speckled rainbow.

1   Make the vinaigrette: In a blender, combine the plum vinegar, rice vinegar, ginger, lime juice, and tamari. With the blender still running, slowly drizzle in the olive oil and sesame oil to emulsify. Set aside.

2   Make the fillings: In a medium saucepot, bring the rice and ½ cup (120 ml) of water to a boil. Reduce to the lowest simmer possible and cover. Cook for 45 minutes. Remove the pot from the heat and let the rice sit for 15 minutes, covered, before transferring the rice to a bowl and tossing it with the sesame oil. Allow the rice to cool.

3   In another medium saucepan, bring the lentils and ¾ cup (180 ml) of water to a boil and cook for 30 minutes, or until the lentils are slightly tender. Drain any excess water.

4   Assemble the wraps: Fill a large, wide bowl with water. Dip a rice paper wrapper in the water for just 2 to 3 seconds. Resist oversoaking—even if the paper is a bit stiff, it will continue to absorb water as you assemble the wrap. Place the paper on a clean work surface.

5 Arrange the rice, lentils, cilantro, avocado, beets, carrots, daikon, and strawberries down the center of the wrappers lengthwise. To roll, carefully fold up one of the short ends of the wrappers over the filling. Then fold one of the longer sides over the toppings and carefully roll the wrap toward the other edge of the wrapper to seal. Repeat with the remaining ingredients. Slice each wrap in half and serve with the ginger-lime vinaigrette for dipping.

Light
WORK ━━━━━━━

DANCE CHALLENGE Practice being bold and not judging yourself. Choose a song you love, one that always boosts your mood. Now turn it on, crank it up, and dance! Doesn't matter where or when; just let it flow. Take a video of yourself dancing, watch it, and send yourself love as you do. Bonus points if you send the video to someone in your trusted circle.

WILD RICE + KIMCHI GRAIN BOWL

⅔ cup (130 g) uncooked
    wild rice

1 tablespoon plus 1 teaspoon
    extra-virgin olive oil

1 tablespoon tamari soy sauce

1 large portobello mushroom,
    wiped clean and stem
    discarded

16 green beans, ends trimmed

½ cup (85 g) cooked or canned
    black beans, rinsed and
    drained

Himalayan salt

6 cups (180 g) baby spinach

½ cup (75 g) kimchi

2 teaspoons hemp seeds

Green Goddess Dressing
    (page 202)

Whole-grain wild rice is one of the most easily digested foods on the planet, is naturally gluten-free, and is rich in protein, thiamine, calcium, magnesium, fiber, and potassium. Here we've paired it up with earthy, meaty portobello mushrooms and fiber-ful green beans, plus gut-powering kimchi and a drizzle of Green Goddess Dressing.

1   In a small pot, combine the rice and 1 cup (240 ml) of water and bring to a boil. Cover the pot and lower the heat to a simmer. Cook for 20 to 30 minutes, or until the rice is tender. If the rice absorbs all the water before it's fully cooked, add a tablespoon or two more of water, cover, and continue cooking. If the rice is fully cooked and hasn't absorbed all the water, simply strain the rice and discard the extra water. Set aside, covered.

2   Preheat the oven to 375°F (190°C). In a medium bowl, whisk together 1 tablespoon of the oil and the tamari. Rub the outside of the mushroom cap with half of the mixture and toss the green beans with the remaining marinade. Arrange the mushroom and green beans on a baking sheet in single layer and roast for 10 minutes. Remove the green beans and roast the mushroom for about 10 more minutes, or until tender and juicy. Cut the mushroom into ½-inch-thick (12 mm) slices and allow them to sit in their juices while you continue to prep.

3   In a medium bowl, toss the black beans with the remaining 1 teaspoon of oil and a pinch of salt. Set aside.

4   Divide the spinach between 2 medium bowls and top each with half of the warm rice. Allow the spinach to wilt for about 5 minutes. Divide the vegetables, beans, and kimchi between the 2 bowls, and give each a sprinkle of hemp seeds and a drizzle of dressing.

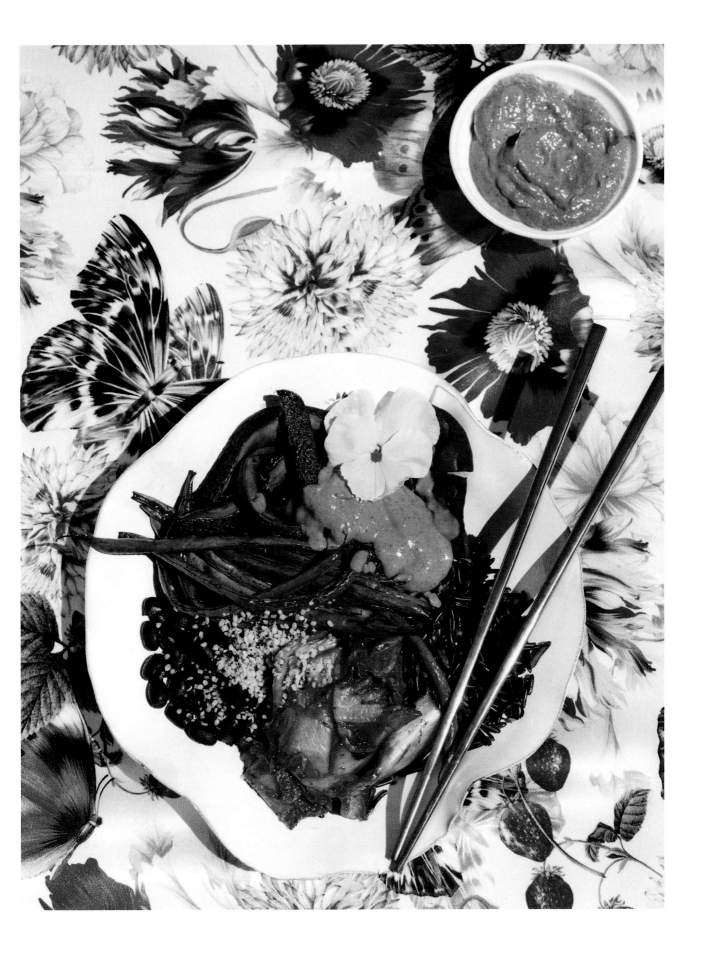

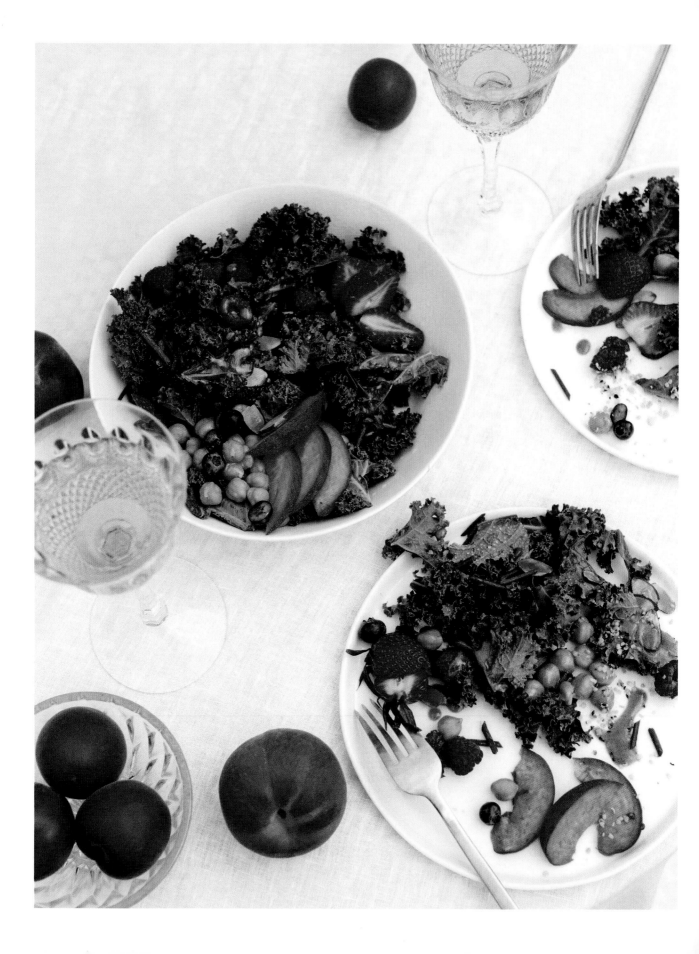

SEXIEST SALAD IN NEW YORK CITY

SERVES 2

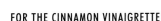

FOR THE CINNAMON VINAIGRETTE

¼ cup (60 ml) sunflower oil

2 tablespoons wildflower honey

2 tablespoons Dijon mustard

3 teaspoons apple cider vinegar

½ teaspoon ground cinnamon

Pinch of Himalayan salt

FOR THE SALAD

¼ cup (25 g) sliced almonds

8 cups (240 g) torn kale leaves

¾ cup (125 g) cooked or canned chickpeas, rinsed and drained

½ cup (95 g) blueberries

½ cup (65 g) raspberries

1 peach, thinly sliced

4 large strawberries, hulled and thinly sliced

¼ cup (12 g) minced chives

2 tablespoons hemp seeds

This salad was designed to make you feel sexy inside and out, and since we're city girls, we decided to name it after our beloved urban jungle. There's nothing more sensual than biting into a sun-ripened peach or berry and having the sweet juice run down your chin as the flavors erupt in your mouth . . . at least there wasn't until we laid berries and a peach atop a bed of cleansing kale and drizzled them with a dressing spiked with cinnamon, a natural aphrodisiac that increases blood circulation while stimulating the metabolism. Disclaimer: We are not responsible for any spontaneous rendezvous or purchases of leopard-print thongs (you too, boys) that may occur while under the influence of this salad.

1   Make the dressing: In a jar or blender, add all the ingredients. Shake or blend until completely smooth. Set aside.

2   Scatter the sliced almonds in a large pan over medium-low heat. Toast the nuts, stirring occasionally, until lightly browned and fragrant, about 5 minutes. Set aside to cool.

3   In 2 medium bowls, make beds with the kale. Top with the chickpeas, blueberries, raspberries, peach, and strawberries. Sprinkle with the chives, hemp seeds, and toasted almonds and drizzle with the dressing.

LUNCH

CREAMY FLAXSEED SALAD

FOR THE FLAXSEED MAYO

1 tablespoon flaxseed meal

3 tablespoons extra-virgin olive
    oil or sunflower oil

1 clove garlic, minced

1 teaspoon Dijon mustard

½ teaspoon Himalayan salt

6 drops stevia

FOR THE SALAD

1 cup (140 g) raw almonds,
    soaked overnight and
    drained

2 stalks celery, finely chopped

2 scallions (white and green
    parts), thinly sliced

½ cup (55 g) goji berries,
    roughly chopped

1 clove garlic, minced

1 teaspoon Dijon mustard

1½ teaspoons fresh lemon juice

¼ teaspoon Himalayan salt, or
    more to taste

Freshly ground black pepper

FOR FINISHING

Pinch of kelp granules, sliced
    cucumber, gluten-free
    bread, crackers, Daily
    Greens (page 33), and
    lemon wedges (optional)

EAT CLEAN

This summery delight features flaked almonds plus hydrating celery for quintessential crunch, and goji berries for subtle sweet bites à la raisins or cranberries. But the true highlight is our homemade flax mayo, which goes head-to-head with any store-bought variety and can be stashed in the fridge to satisfy all your sandwich, wrap, dip, or dressing desires. (Dress it up with garlic, hot sauce, curry, or any other spice and seasoning your heart calls for.)

1   Make the mayo: In a small pot, combine the flaxseed meal with 3 tablespoons of water over medium heat. Stirring constantly, heat the mixture gently until it has thickened, about 2 minutes. Remove the mixture from the heat and allow it to cool to room temperature.

2   In a blender, combine the flax mixture with 1 tablespoon of the oil. Blend on high for 15 to 20 seconds. Scrape down the sides of the blender with a spatula, add 1 tablespoon of the oil, and blend for another 15 seconds. Repeat this a third time, making sure all the oil is incorporated before adding the remaining 1 tablespoon of oil. The mixture should be thick and white like mayo.

3   Add the garlic, mustard, salt, and stevia and blend again. Set aside.

4   Make the salad: Add the almonds to a food processor and process until finely chopped. Transfer to a medium mixing bowl and add the celery, scallions, berries, garlic, mustard, lemon juice, salt, and a few cracks of black pepper. Stir to combine. Fold in the flaxseed mayo and stir well to combine. Taste and adjust the seasoning, if desired, with more salt or pepper or a pinch of kelp granules.

5   Serve dolloped on cucumber slices, bread, crackers, or greens with lemon wedges, if using.

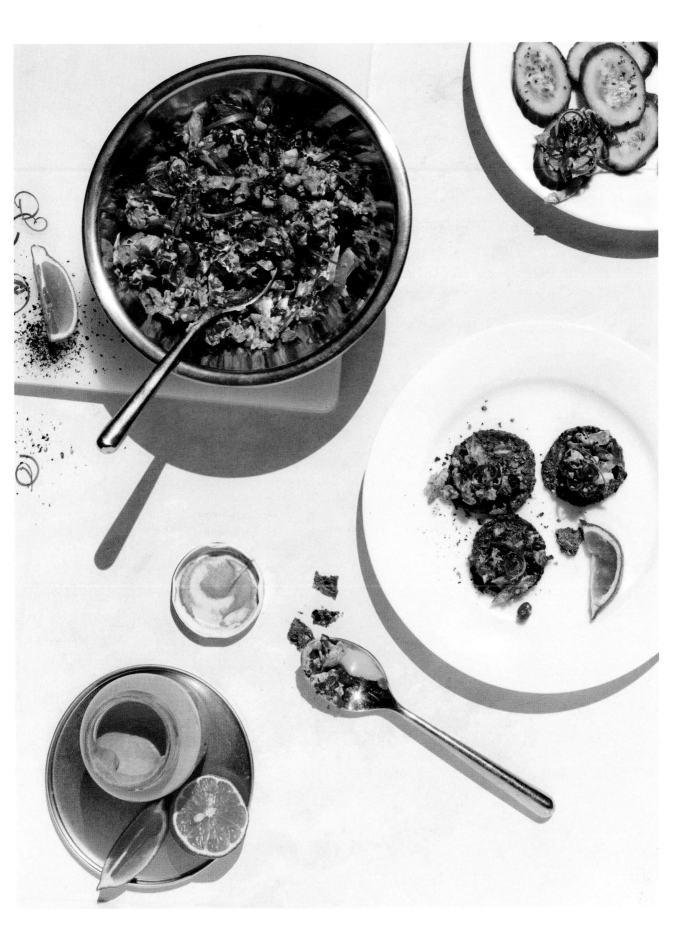

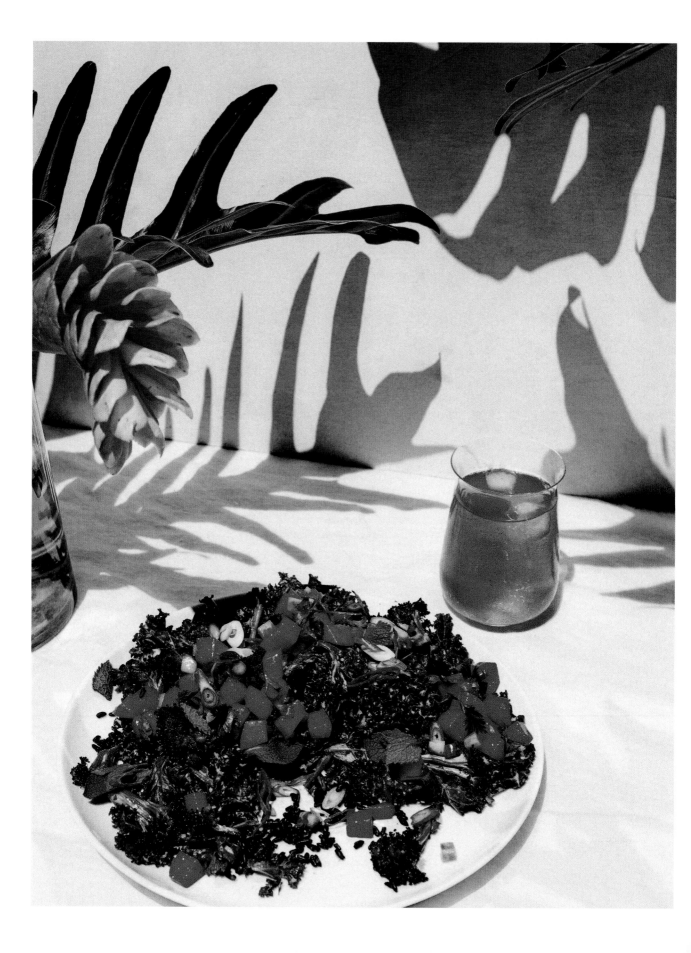

TROPICAL SALAD WITH FORBIDDEN RICE

SERVES 4

FOR THE SALAD

1 cup (200 g) forbidden rice

Himalayan salt

2 scallions (white and green parts), thinly sliced

1 large or 2 small heads broccoli, broken up into bite-size florets

2 teaspoons extra-virgin olive oil

FOR THE MANGO SALSA

1 tablespoon wildflower honey

1 tablespoon fresh lime juice

2 teaspoons extra-virgin olive oil

½ teaspoon Himalayan salt

2 fresh mangoes, cut into ½-inch (12 mm) cubes

1 cucumber, cut into ¼-inch (6 mm) cubes

1 medium shallot, minced

8 sprigs fresh cilantro, leaves roughly chopped

4 sprigs fresh mint, leaves picked and torn

FOR FINISHING

8 cups (540 g) curly kale, chopped (about 2 bunches)

Jalapeño + Tahini Dressing (page 202)

We don't love forbidden rice just for its sexy purple-black color—we're particularly enamored because, of all the rices, it is the richest in disease-fighting antioxidants, fiber, and anti-inflammatory properties. We've paired this ancient grain with mango salsa and spicy jalapeño–tahini dressing for a warm-weather getaway in a bowl.

1 Preheat the oven to 350°F (175°C).

2 Make the salad: In a small pot, bring the rice and 1½ cups (360 ml) of water to a boil with a pinch of salt. Cover, reduce the heat to low, and let the rice simmer for 30 minutes, or until it has absorbed all the water. Turn off the heat and let the rice rest for 5 minutes before fluffing it with a fork and folding in the scallions. Season to taste with salt and set aside to cool.

3 In a large bowl, toss the broccoli with the oil and a pinch of salt. Spread the broccoli evenly over a baking sheet and roast for 15 minutes, or until the broccoli is tender. Set aside.

4 Make the mango salsa: In a medium bowl, whisk together the honey, lime juice, oil, and salt. Add the mango, cucumber, shallot, cilantro, and mint and toss to coat with the lime juice mixture.

5 Assemble the salad: In a large bowl, drizzle the kale with enough dressing to coat and gently massage the dressing into the greens until just tender. Fold in the roasted broccoli with a bit more dressing. Top the kale with the rice and the mango salsa. Serve with additional dressing, if desired.

YOUTH + BEAUTY SALAD

FOR THE PUMPKIN SEED AND LEMON DRESSING

¼ cup (60 ml) fresh lemon juice

½ cup (120 ml) raw pumpkin seed oil

1 teaspoon grated fresh ginger

2 cloves garlic, minced

Himalayan salt and freshly ground black pepper

FOR THE SALAD

1 head romaine lettuce, or your favorite gem variety, chopped into 1-inch (2.5 cm) strips

1 large beet, sliced into matchsticks

1 cucumber, sliced into matchsticks

4 small carrots, sliced into matchsticks

8 radishes, sliced into matchsticks

2 bunches fresh mint, leaves picked

1 cup (175 g) pomegranate seeds

¼ cup (35 g) raw pumpkin seeds

¼ cup (35 g) sunflower seeds

¼ cup (40 g) hemp seeds

This is the ultimate age-fighting, ultrahydrating beauty-in-a-bowl salad, specifically designed to enhance your natural beauty from the inside out. Cucumbers nourish your cells, beets and carrots bring a healthy color to your cheeks, and pomegranates deliver antioxidants and keep signs of aging at bay while greens help eliminate toxins and add an extra dose of hydration for a Sakara glow. It's all sealed with a superfood kiss of vitamin E–rich hemp seeds for skin plumping and chia for strong, glossy hair. Nurture your best self and your shining spirit will radiate your inner beauty outward.

1   Make the dressing: In a blender, combine all the ingredients with a pinch of salt and a couple of cracks of pepper and blend until smooth. Season with more salt and pepper to taste.

2   Make the salad: Divide the lettuce among 4 large or 6 medium salad bowls. Top with the beet, cucumber, carrots, and radishes, then with the mint and pomegranate seeds.

3   In a small bowl, combine the pumpkin, sunflower, and hemp seeds and sprinkle the mixture over the top of each bowl. Finish off the salads with a drizzle of dressing.

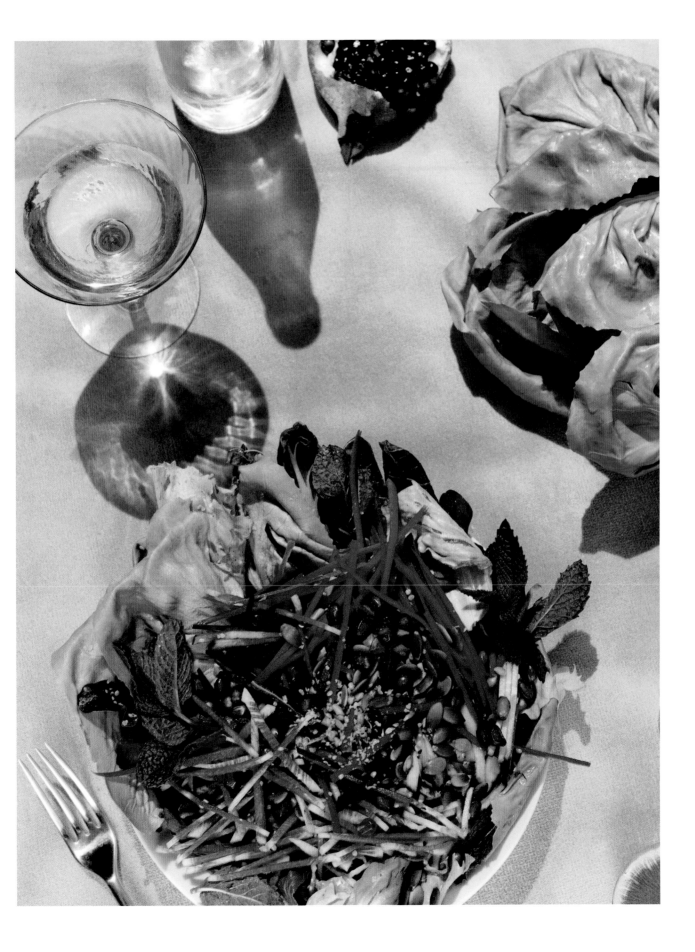

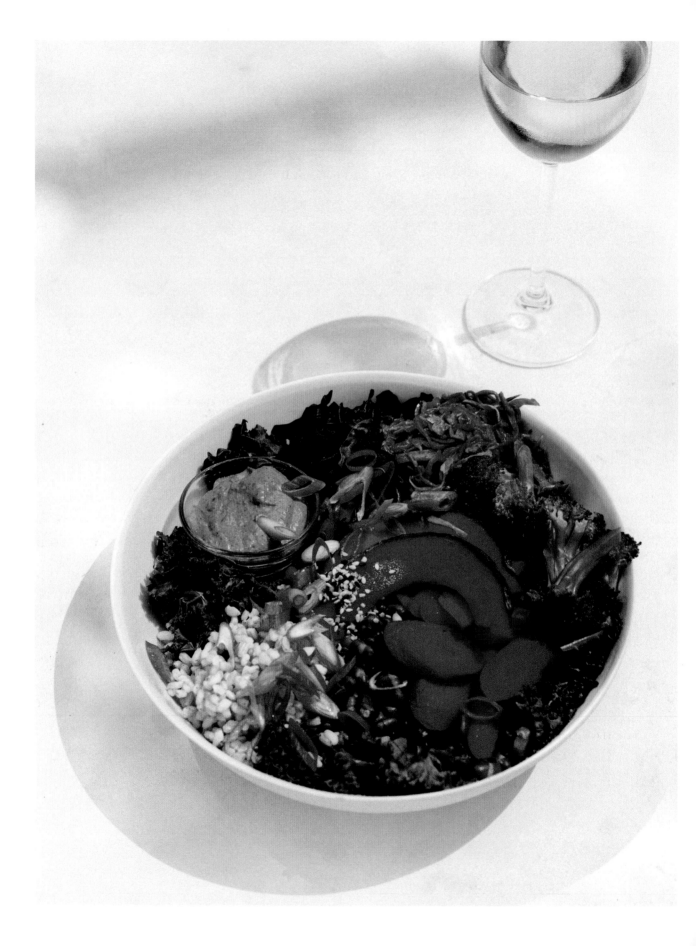

BALANCING MACRO PLATE

This is one of our go-to dishes. It's one of the most potent tools we have in our dietary toolbox because it's a powerful fix for bringing the body back into balance (and keeping it there). Macrobiotics, or a philosophy of eating that draws on Zen Buddhism, is all about achieving equilibrium and harmony in the body, which in turn leads to boosted health, boosted moods, boosted feelings of connection—an all-around life boost. The key macro components are a balanced lineup of simple cooked veggies, whole grains, legumes, and sea vegetables. Balance is something that we strive for in our Sakara meals and also in life.

SERVES 4

FOR THE MARINATED CABBAGE

2 cups (200 g) shredded purple cabbage

2 tablespoons extra-virgin olive oil

¼ cup (60 ml) red wine vinegar

¼ teaspoon Himalayan salt

FOR THE VEGETABLES

½ butternut or kabocha squash, cut into thin slices

3 large carrots, sliced into 1-inch (2.5 cm) pieces

2 cups (350 g) broccoli florets

12 cups (810 g) chopped curly kale (about 3 heads)

FOR THE TAHINI-AVOCADO DRESSING

1 cup (100 g) fresh cilantro leaves, roughly chopped

½ avocado, pitted and peeled

⅓ cup (10 g) packed baby spinach

3 tablespoons tahini

2 tablespoons apple cider vinegar

2 tablespoons olive oil

2 cloves garlic, peeled

1 tablespoon fresh lemon juice

½ teaspoon Himalayan salt

¼ teaspoon freshly ground black pepper

FOR FINISHING

2 cups (500 g) cooked brown rice

1 cup (230 g) cooked or canned adzuki beans, rinsed and drained

¼ cup (6 g) hijiki seaweed, soaked for 15 minutes and drained

3 scallions (white and green parts), thinly sliced

2 tablespoons sesame seeds

RECIPE CONTINUES

95

1   Make the marinated cabbage: In a medium bowl, toss the cabbage with the oil, vinegar, and salt. Allow the cabbage to marinate overnight in the fridge. Drain the cabbage before serving.

2   Make the vegetables: In a large pot fitted with a steamer basket, bring 1 to 2 inches (2.5 to 6 cm) of water to a boil and reduce to a simmer. Add the squash and steam, covered, until fork-tender, about 10 minutes. Remove the squash and add the carrots. Steam until fork-tender, about 10 minutes. Remove the carrots and add the broccoli. Steam until tender, 3 to 5 minutes. Remove the broccoli and add the kale. Steam until bright green and just tender, 2 to 3 minutes. Set the vegetables aside to cool.

3   Make the dressing: In a blender, combine all the ingredients with ¼ cup (60 ml) plus 2 tablespoons of water and blend until smooth. Add more water to loosen the consistency, if desired. Taste and adjust the seasoning, if needed.

4   Serve: Divide each of the components among 4 large serving bowls: start with a bed of steamed greens, followed by the rice, beans, steamed squash, carrots, and broccoli, and the hijiki. Top with the marinated cabbage, a sprinkling of scallions and sesame seeds, and a drizzle of dressing. Store any leftover dressing in the fridge for up to 3 days.

SEA VEGETABLES

Sea vegetables ARE SOME OF THE MOST *beautifying foods* ON THE PLANET

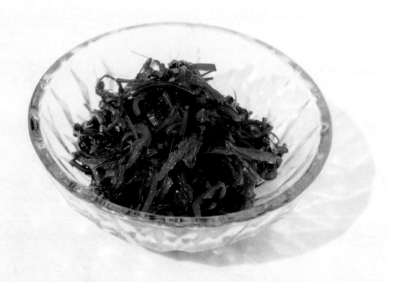

Sea vegetables, or seaweeds like hijiki, dulse, wakame, or nori, are particularly great for the skin and infuse the entire body with vitamins, protein, fiber, omega-3s, and essential minerals like potassium, iron, and calcium. They help rid the body of disease-causing heavy metals and reduce water retention (see ya, cellulite!) while improving circulation, oxygenating the body, and aiding digestion. And they're an amazing source of iodine, which keeps the thyroid balanced and healthy. Sea vegetables also add a naturally salty and from-the-sea umami flavor to any dish. Throw some hijiki or dulse into salads, add wakame or kombu to soups and broths, or roll up anything and everything in a sheet of nori.

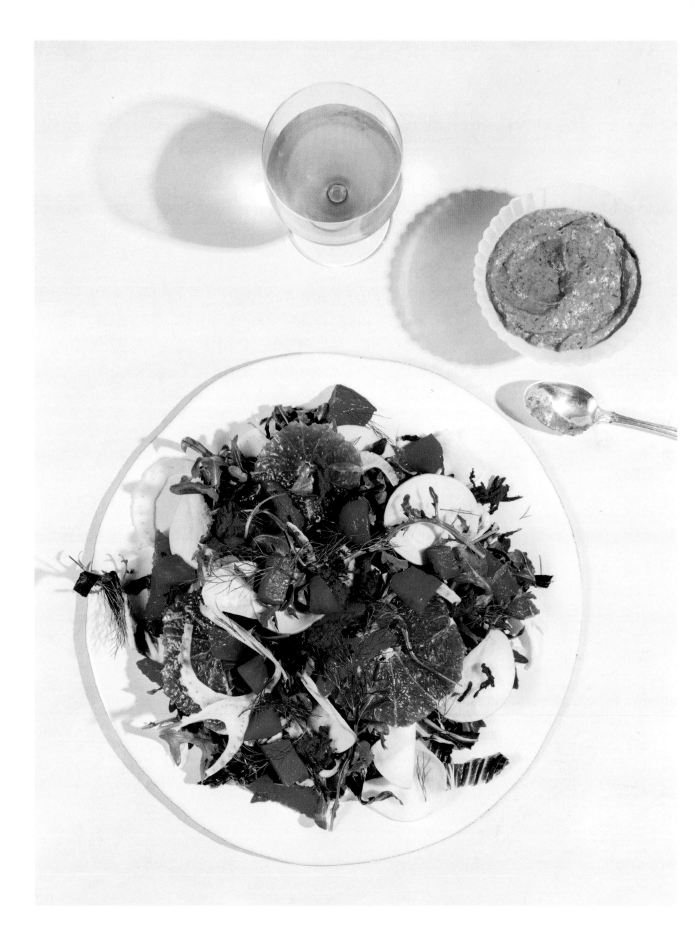

CITRUS DETOX SALAD

A little bitterness is a good thing—at least in your greens. Leafy plants that bite back, such as mustard greens, dandelion greens, and arugula, are one of the most cleansing, balancing foods you can deliver to your body. They stimulate the liver, helping it better absorb nutrients and perform its detoxifying duties (which in turn keeps hormones balanced and metabolizes fats); flush out unnecessary fluids; purify the blood; and keep your skin clear. These greens also jump-start enzyme production in the digestive tract, which assists in breaking down foods more effectively and efficiently. That means more nutrient absorption for you and fewer wasted resources for your plants. And, in Ayurveda, it's recommended that you enjoy each of the flavors—sweet, salty, sour, bitter, pungent, and astringent—in order to keep the body in balanced harmony.

SERVES 4

FOR THE CARROT CRISPS

2 teaspoons extra-virgin olive oil

½ cup (30 g) nutritional yeast

2 teaspoons ground flaxseeds

1 teaspoon chia seeds

¼ teaspoon ground turmeric

¼ teaspoon Himalayan salt, or more to taste

Small pinch of cayenne pepper

2 large carrots, peeled and grated, excess liquid drained

1 tablespoon fresh lemon juice

FOR THE MARINATED BEETS

2 medium golden beets, scrubbed

3 tablespoons extra-virgin olive oil

½ teaspoon Himalayan salt, or more to taste

¼ cup (60 ml) brown rice vinegar

¼ cup (60 ml) fresh-squeezed orange juice

2 tablespoons lemon juice

2 tablespoons wildflower honey

FOR THE SALAD

2 cups (110 g) dandelion greens

2 cups (80 g) radicchio

8 cups (160 g) arugula

4 small baby turnips, thinly sliced (a mandoline is nice here)

1 small bulb fennel, thinly sliced (ditto on the mandoline), fronds reserved

1 grapefruit

1 orange

Green Citrus Dressing (page 204)

RECIPE CONTINUES

1   Make the carrot crisps: Preheat the oven to 350°F (175°C). Line a baking sheet with parchment paper and lightly brush the parchment with olive oil. Set aside.

2   In a blender or spice grinder, combine the yeast, flaxseeds, chia seeds, turmeric, salt, and cayenne. Grind until the mixture is a fine powder. In a large bowl, combine the grated carrot with the lemon juice and toss to coat. Add the powder and toss again until everything is thoroughly mixed. Spread the mixture evenly across the baking sheet and bake for 30 minutes. Give the mixture a toss and continue baking for another 30 minutes, or until the carrots are lightly browned and crisped. Let the mixture cool before using your hands to create a crumble. Set aside.

3   Make the marinated beets: Preheat the oven to 400°F (205°C).

4   Arrange the beets on a baking sheet and drizzle them with 1 tablespoon of the oil. Add a sprinkle of salt and rub the beets to coat. Roast for 40 to 50 minutes, or until you can easily slide a paring knife through them. Allow the beets to cool until they're comfortable to handle.

5   In a medium bowl, whisk together the remaining 2 tablespoons of oil, the salt, vinegar, orange juice, lemon juice, and honey and set aside.

6   Once the beets have cooled, use your fingers to gently slip off the skins. Cut the beets into ½-inch (12 mm) pieces and place them in a large bowl. Toss the beets with the vinaigrette and let them marinate for at least 30 minutes, or as long as overnight (they get tastier the longer they sit).

7   Assemble the salad: Roughly chop the dandelion greens into bite-size pieces and add them to a large bowl. Quarter the radicchio, cut the wedges into thick ribbons, and add them to the bowl. Sprinkle in the arugula, turnips, and fennel and use your hands to give everything a toss.

8   To segment the grapefruit, slice the top and bottom off the fruit so it sits steadily on your cutting board. Follow the curve of the fruit with your knife to slice off the skin and white pith. Gently slice into the fruit between the white membranes to remove the segments. Repeat with the orange.

9   Divide the lettuce mixture among 4 plates. Top with marinated beets, grapefruit and orange segments, a small handful of the carrot crunch, and a drizzle of dressing. Garnish each plate with the fennel fronds.

Light WORK

LOVE YOURSELF This challenge is about changing the way you talk to yourself. Write yourself a note with the following mantra: "I am strong, powerful, and beautiful. I love my body, and my body loves me." Tape the note to your mirror. Each morning, when you look in the mirror, instead of criticizing your perceived imperfections, repeat the mantra. Know it and believe it!

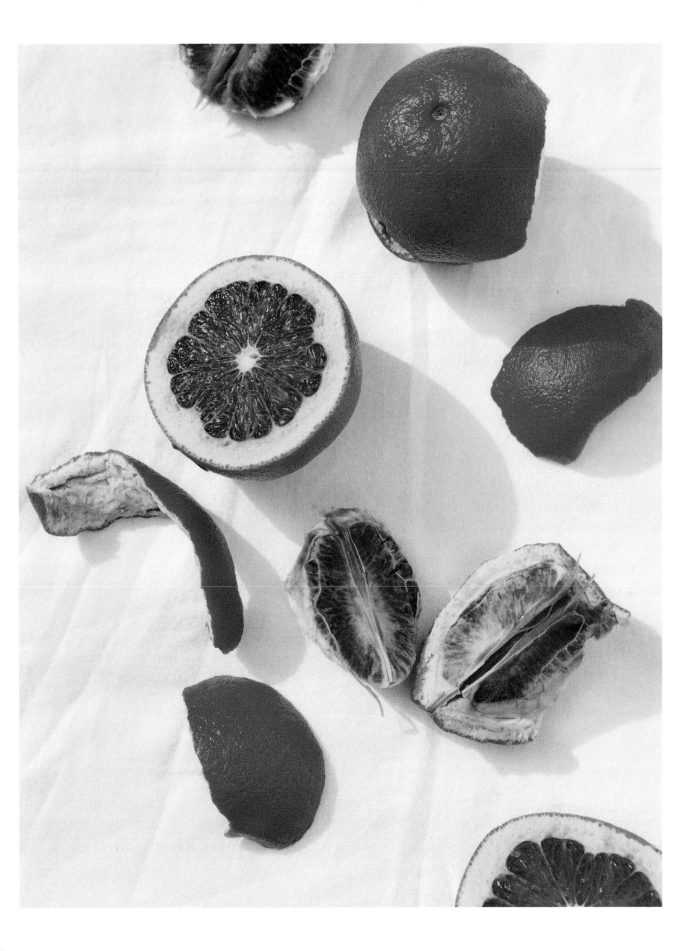

CLEOPATRA'S CAULIFLOWER SALAD

Cleopatra was well versed in superfoods and regularly called upon natural healers like oats, hemp, honey, and sea salt as part of her health and beauty routine. As a nod to the food traditions and wisdom of Egypt, we've embraced a few of Queen Cleo's favorites in this salad. Most notably, we've adorned this dish with dukkah, a flavorful blend of hazelnuts and herbs. A key ingredient in traditional dukkah is coriander, a curative plant whose healing power is almost as epic as its history. Egyptians placed these little seeds in their tombs as sacred offerings that symbolized enduring love. Coriander's reputation has endured too—modern science has found that it has potent antibacterial properties and can help settle the stomach and stimulate digestion. We've added hemp seeds to the mix because, as Cleopatra knew, these (non-psychoactive) seeds from the *Cannabis sativa* plant are essential plant medicine. Hemp seeds are exceedingly rich in two essential fatty acids, linoleic acid (an omega-6) and alpha-linolenic acid (an omega-3); are a significant source of protein (more than 25 percent of their total calories are from high-quality protein); and abound in vitamin E and minerals. These potent seeds nourish the skin, charge up the immune system, aid digestion, and offer the body a supercharged alternative fuel source. Sprinkled over roasted sulfur-rich cauliflower (we especially love the jewel-toned purple variety), juicy peaches, and a citrus-herb chermoula, this dukkah makes for a salad fit for royalty.

RECIPE CONTINUES

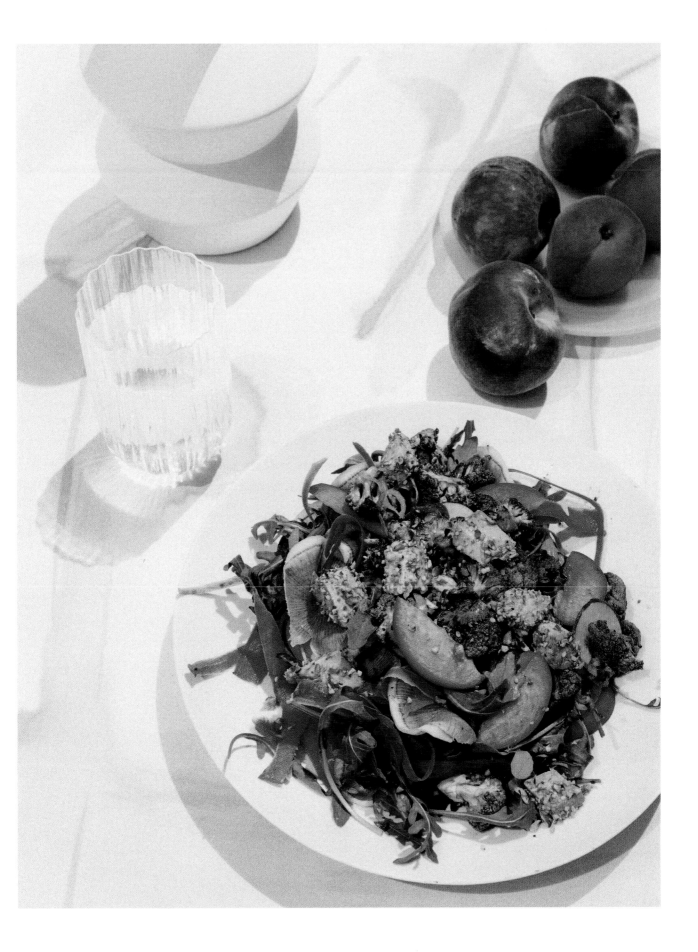

FOR THE ROASTED CAULIFLOWER

1 head cauliflower, broken up into bite-size florets

1 large shallot, sliced into thin rings

2 tablespoons extra-virgin olive oil

½ teaspoon Himalayan salt

FOR THE CHERMOULA

6 sprigs fresh cilantro, stems and leaves chopped into 1-inch (2.5 cm) pieces

3 sprigs fresh parsley, leaves picked

2 small cloves garlic, sliced

1 teaspoon Himalayan salt

½ teaspoon ground cumin

¼ teaspoon smoked paprika

Dash of cayenne pepper

Juice of 1 lemon

¼ cup (60 ml) extra-virgin olive oil

FOR THE HEMP-DUKKAH TOPPING

2 tablespoons roughly chopped toasted hazelnuts

2 tablespoons hemp seeds

2 teaspoons sesame seeds

¼ teaspoon ground cumin

¼ teaspoon ground coriander

Freshly ground black pepper

FOR THE SALAD

8 cups (160 g) packed arugula

4 radishes, halved and sliced into thin half-moons

1 peach, sliced

1 medium carrot, shaved into ribbons with a vegetable peeler or grated

1 avocado, pitted and diced into 1-inch (2.5 cm) cubes

2 teaspoons extra-virgin olive oil

Juice of 1 lemon

2 tablespoons dried cranberries

1   Make the roasted cauliflower: Preheat the oven to 375°F (190°C). Line a baking sheet with parchment paper and set aside.

2   In a large bowl, toss together the cauliflower and shallot with the oil and salt. Arrange the vegetables on the prepared baking sheet and roast for 20 minutes, or until the cauliflower and shallots are brown, tender, and a bit crispy. Set aside to cool.

3   Make the chermoula: In a food processor, combine the cilantro, parsley, garlic, salt, cumin, paprika, cayenne pepper, and lemon juice and pulse until the mixture is coarsely chopped. Scrape down the sides of the bowl with a rubber spatula and, with the food processor running, slowly stream in the oil. Process until the sauce is mostly smooth. Pour the chermoula over the cauliflower and shallot mixture and set aside.

4   Make the hemp-dukkah topping: In a small bowl, combine all the ingredients with a few cracks of black pepper. Set aside.

5   Assemble the salad: In a large bowl, toss together the arugula, radishes, peach, carrot, and avocado with the oil and lemon juice. Divide the mixture between 2 bowls and top each with half of the dressed cauliflower and shallots, hemp-dukkah topping, cranberries, and any remaining chermoula left in the bottom of the bowl.

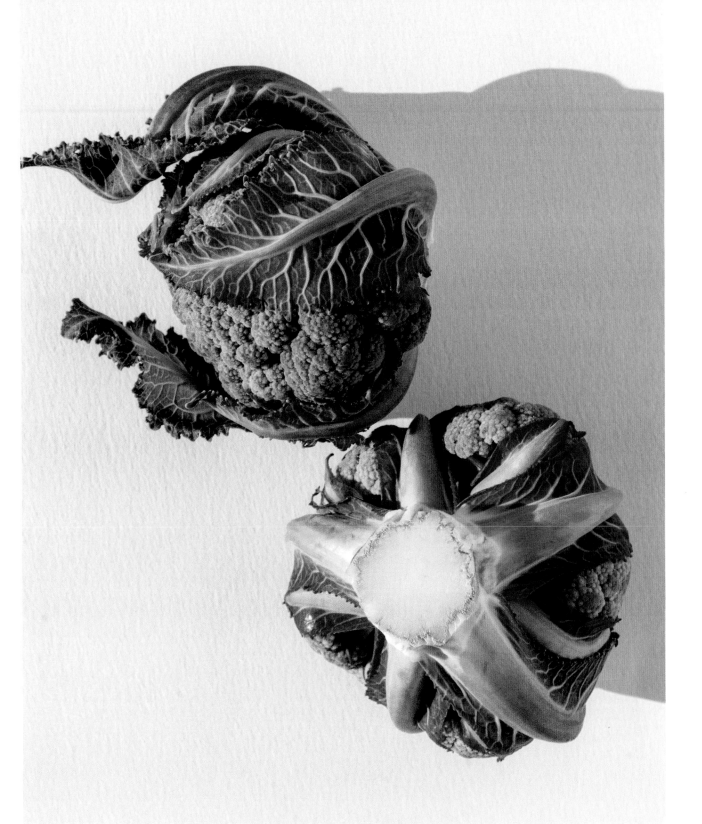

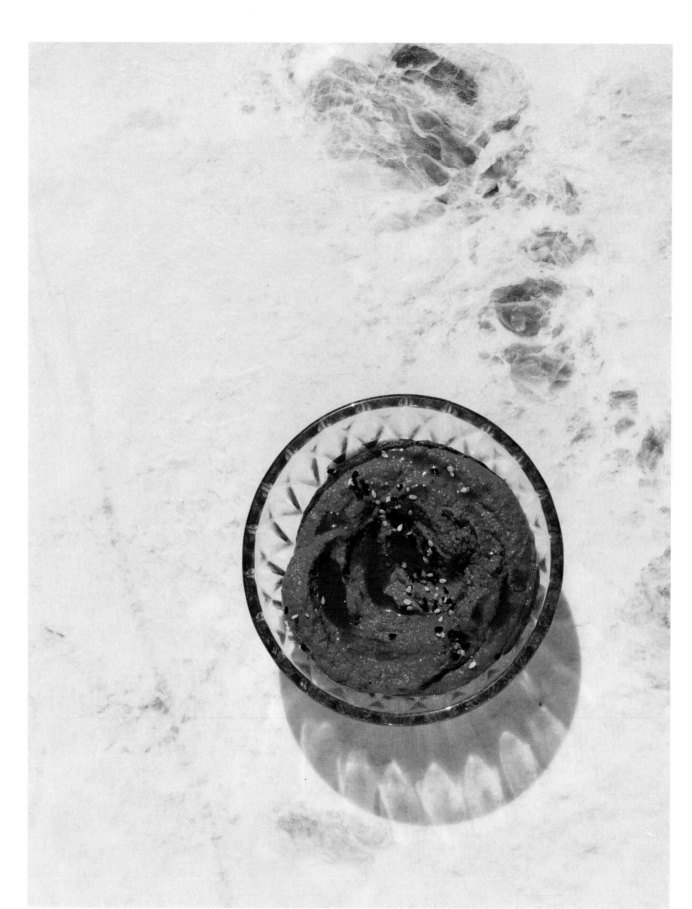

PINK BEET HUMMUS

**MAKES ABOUT
3 CUPS (720 ML)**

1 pound (.4 kg) red beets
(about 2 medium)

1 tablespoon plus 1 teaspoon
extra-virgin olive oil

1 teaspoon Himalayan salt, or
more to taste

1 cup (165 g) cooked or canned
chickpeas, rinsed and
drained

¼ cup (60 ml) tahini

3 tablespoons fresh lemon juice

2 cloves garlic, roughly
chopped

Freshly ground black pepper

1 tablespoon black and white
sesame seeds, for garnish
(optional)

The color pink is a universal symbol of love, nurturing, and kindness, and this charmingly rosy dip is no exception. By adding red beets into the mix, we give traditional hummus an antioxidant-infused makeover that's as beautiful on the plate as it is in the body. Spread this over wraps, whisk it into dressings, or pair it with market finds for a simple crudité. Whatever you choose, serve it with heart.

1   Preheat the oven to 400°F (205°C).

2   Scrub the beets, drizzle them with 1 teaspoon of the oil, and sprinkle with a pinch of salt. Arrange them on a baking sheet and roast for 40 to 50 minutes, or until you can easily pierce them with a knife. Allow the beets to cool completely, then use your hands to gently slip off their skins.

3   Roughly chop the beets and add them to a food processor along with the chickpeas, tahini, lemon juice, garlic, and a few cracks of pepper. Add ¼ cup (60 ml) of water and process until very smooth, adding more water if you'd like a thinner hummus. Store in the fridge for up to 1 week. Garnish with sesame seeds, if desired.

LUNCH

ROASTED RADISH + TURMERIC-GINGER BOWL

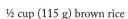

½ cup (115 g) brown rice

2 large carrots, cut into 1-inch (2.5 cm) rounds

8 radishes, halved

4 teaspoons extra-virgin olive oil

½ teaspoon sesame seeds

½ teaspoon red pepper flakes

Himalayan salt

½ cucumber, peeled, halved lengthwise, and sliced into ½-inch (2.5 cm) half-moons

Juice of 1 lemon

1 teaspoon toasted sesame oil

1 teaspoon hemp seeds

6 cups (180 g) spinach

Ginger + Turmeric Dressing (page 204)

We love ginger for its spicy, aromatic allure. It is high in gingerol—a compound with powerful anti-inflammatory and antioxidant benefits that can also fight infection—and can help reduce muscle pain and soreness, lower blood sugar levels, improve heart disease risk factors, reduce LDL cholesterol and blood triglyceride levels, prevent age-related damage to the brain, and—major bonus—relieve discomfort during the menstrual cycle.

1   Preheat the oven to 375°F (190°C). Cover a baking sheet with parchment paper or foil and set aside.

2   Bring the rice and 1 cup (240 ml) of water to a boil in a small saucepan. Reduce to a simmer and cook for 30 minutes, or until the rice is tender and the water has evaporated. If all the water has evaporated and the rice is not yet cooked, add a couple of tablespoons of water and continue cooking until tender.

3   In a medium bowl, toss the carrots and radishes with 2 teaspoons of the olive oil, sesame seeds, red pepper flakes, and a small pinch of salt. Roast on the baking sheet for 20 minutes, or until the vegetables are tender and starting to caramelize. Set aside to cool.

4   In another medium bowl, combine the cucumber, lemon juice, sesame oil, and hemp seeds. Season with salt to taste. Set aside.

5   In a large sauté pan, heat the remaining 2 teaspoons of olive oil over medium-low heat. Add the spinach and a small pinch of salt. Use tongs or a large spoon to gently toss the spinach until it just beings to wilt, about 3 minutes.

6   Serve: Mound the rice and greens side by side in the bottom of a large serving bowl. Heap with the dressed cucumbers and roasted vegetables and drizzle with dressing.

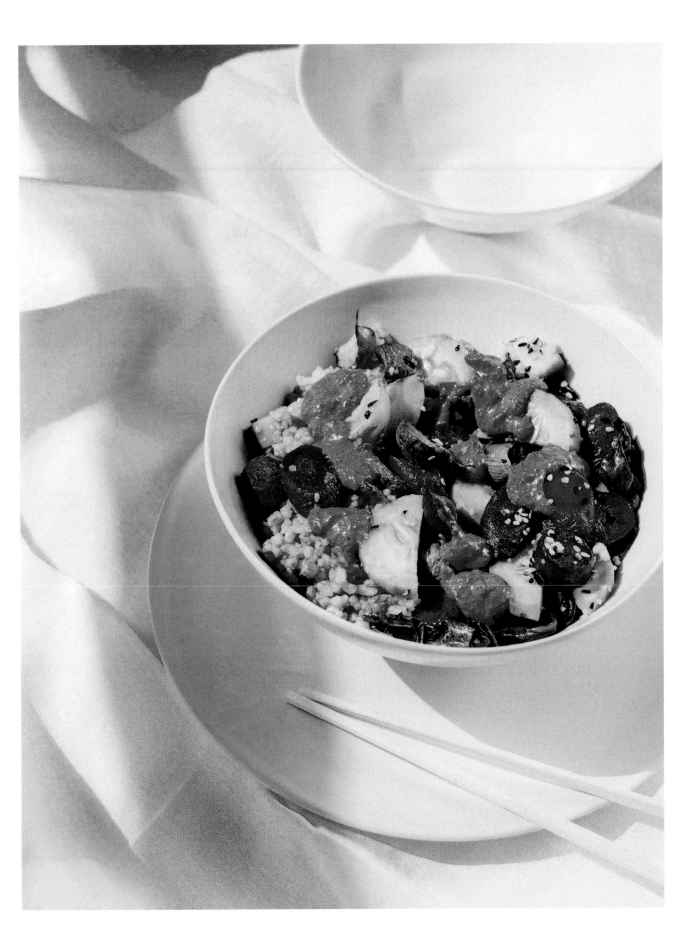

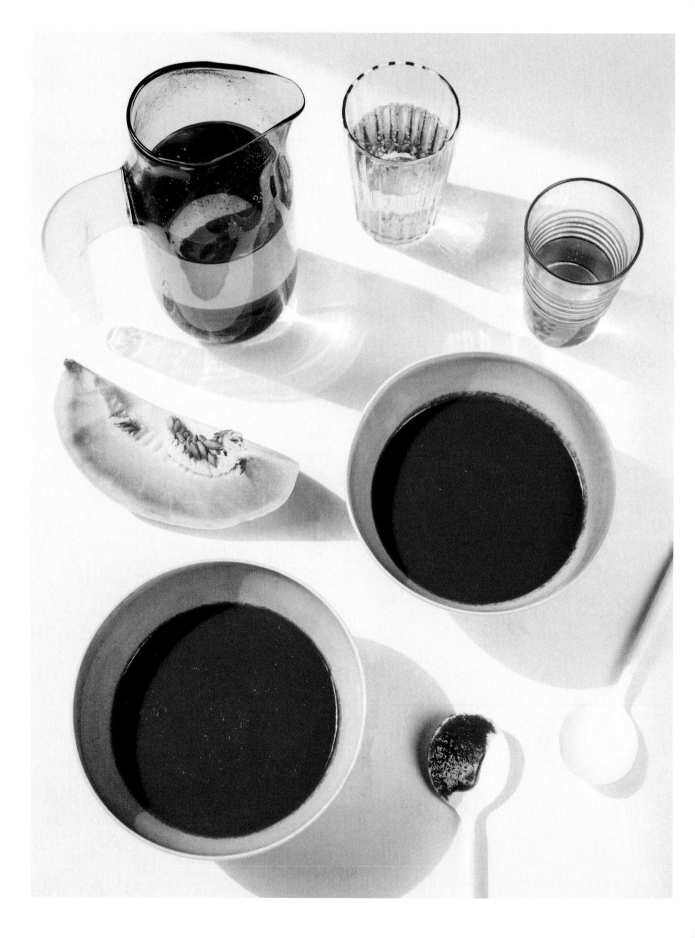

HYDRATING HONEYDEW MELON GAZPACHO

SERVES 2

½ English cucumber, roughly chopped

1 stalk celery, roughly chopped

¼ cup (45 g) honeydew melon, roughly chopped

1 small green tomato, roughly chopped

1 packed cup (30 g) spinach

1 teaspoon lemon juice

1 teaspoon lime juice

1 teaspoon extra-virgin olive oil

6 basil leaves

½ small shallot, roughly chopped

2 tablespoons coconut yogurt or coconut milk

Pinch of Himalayan salt

We developed this soup as a simple and delicious way to nourish your body—particularly your skin—from the inside out. Thanks to its high water content (about 90 percent!), melon is particularly great for flooding your body with H_2O—as are cucumber, celery, and, of course, greens. And spinach (like all dark leafy greens) promotes collagen production and tissue repair while defending the skin with its antioxidant properties from agents that actively break down collagen. It's our secret recipe for a glowing, radiant complexion. We recommend enjoying this soup, whether you're sipping on the go or settling in for a slower, more mindful meal, with a big bowl of Daily Greens (page 33).

In a blender or food processor, combine all the ingredients and blend until smooth. Enjoy right away, or chill before sipping (we like how the flavors come together as it sits). Store in the fridge for up to 3 days.

DAYDREAMER SOBA NOODLE BOWL

SERVES 4

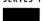

FOR THE CHILI SAUCE

¼ cup (60 ml) plus 2
   tablespoons tahini

3 tablespoons brown rice
   vinegar

2 tablespoons white miso

2 tablespoons tamari soy sauce

1½ tablespoons high-quality
   sriracha

FOR THE NOODLES

2 cups (250 g) shiitake
   mushrooms, stemmed

1 bunch asparagus, woody ends
   trimmed and cut into bite-
   size pieces

1 tablespoon plus 1 teaspoon
   extra-virgin olive oil

½ teaspoon Himalayan salt

1 (12-ounce/340 g) package
   buckwheat soba noodles

4 cups (120 g) baby arugula

2 scallions (white and green
   parts), thinly sliced

1 tablespoon white sesame
   seeds

This masterpiece was dreamed up by one of our chefs who got his start in the world-renowned kitchens of Jean-Georges and Le Bernardin. But the real magic started happening when he applied that fine dining culinary expertise to plant-powered goodness. The result is a dish that is a Sakara mainstay and a longtime client favorite. It's no wonder—it features grounding shiitake mushrooms to keep you focused and connected to the moment, asparagus for cellular regeneration and fortitude, and a fiery chili sauce to ignite your wildest daydreams.

1   Make the chili sauce: In a blender, combine all the ingredients. With the blender still running, drizzle in 2 tablespoons of water to emulsify. Set aside.

2   Make the noodles: Preheat the oven to 350°F (175°C). Line a baking sheet with parchment paper and set aside.

3   In a large bowl, combine the mushrooms and asparagus with 1 tablespoon of the oil and the salt and toss to coat. Spread the vegetables in an even layer over the prepared baking sheet. Roast until the asparagus is tender, about 6 minutes. Transfer the asparagus to a plate and return the mushrooms to the oven to roast for another 10 minutes, until tender. Set aside.

4   Bring a large pot of water to a boil and cook the soba noodles according to the package instructions. Strain and rinse under cold water. Toss the noodles with the remaining 1 teaspoon of oil to keep them from sticking.

5   In a large bowl, toss the noodles with the roasted vegetables and chili sauce. Arrange the noodles over a bed of arugula, sprinkle with the scallions and sesame seeds, and serve.

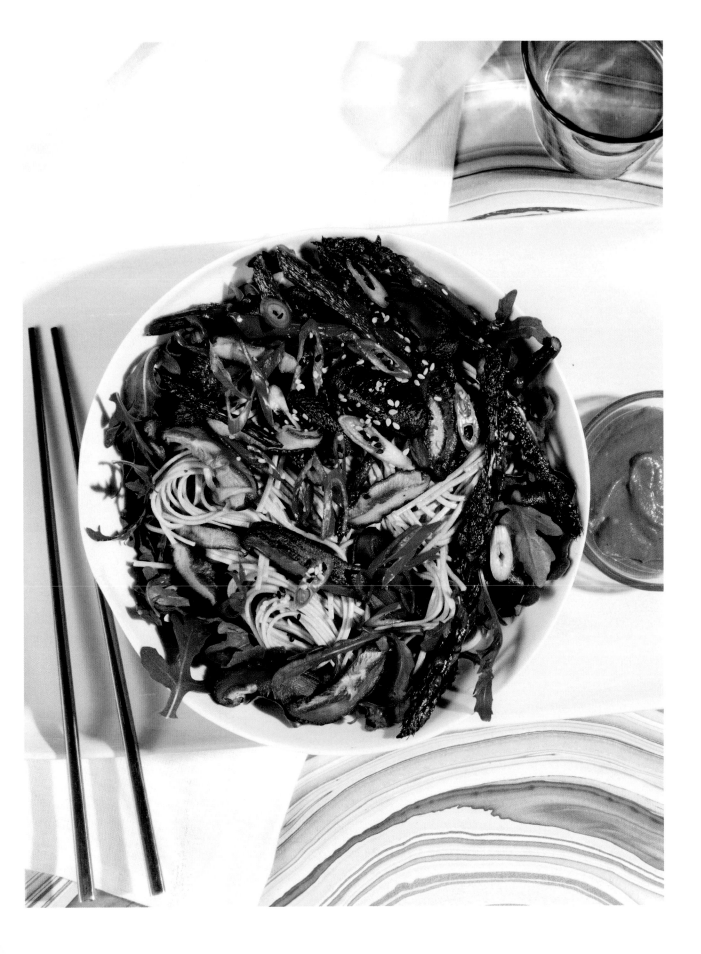

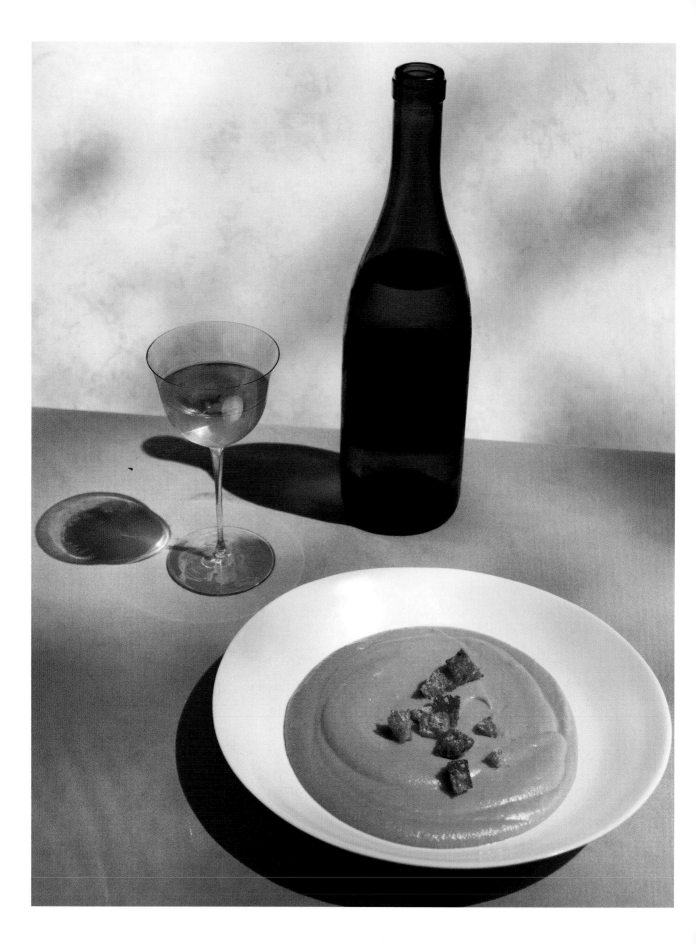

Dinner

Cooking is a time to tune in to your senses, work with your hands, and connect to nature through the bounty of the earth. Whether you're in the mood for something warm and comforting or a fresh and bright salad, to share with friends and loved ones or to eat on your own, be sure to take a moment to have gratitude.

CREAMY CAULIFLOWER SOUP, *following page*

CREAMY CAULIFLOWER SOUP

Did you know that one serving of cauliflower contains *77 percent* of the recommended daily value of vitamin C? It's also a significant source of vitamin K (which helps produce new, healthy bone tissue), magnesium (for healthy bones and teeth, energy production, and general detoxification), folate (to help synthesize and repair DNA), and vitamin B_6 (protector of the immune system and contributor to serotonin production). If that wasn't enough to make this one of our most beloved plants, then consider the alchemy that occurs when cauliflower gets simmered in a flavorful broth and pureed—it becomes silky smooth and oh-so-creamy, as the perfect soup should be. We're always sure to top ours with easy garlic croutons, making this dish just as suitable for a cozy night for two as for a polished evening for ten.

SERVES 4

FOR THE GARLIC CROUTONS

2 (1-inch-thick/2.5 cm) slices Sakara Seed Bread (page 187) or gluten-free bread, cut into ½-inch (12 mm) cubes

1 clove garlic, minced

1 tablespoon extra-virgin olive oil

Pinch of Himalayan salt

FOR THE CAULIFLOWER SOUP

1 tablespoon extra-virgin olive oil, plus more for serving

1 small onion, finely diced

1 clove garlic, minced

¼ cup (30 g) cashews, soaked overnight and drained

4 sprigs fresh thyme, leaves picked

2 teaspoons Himalayan salt, or more to taste

¼ teaspoon smoked paprika

⅛ teaspoon ground turmeric

1 small carrot, grated

1 small head cauliflower, broken up into florets

3 tablespoons nutritional yeast

1   Make the croutons: Preheat the oven to 350°F (175°C).

2   In a medium bowl, combine the bread cubes, garlic, and oil and toss until the bread is evenly coated. Sprinkle the salt on top and toss once more. Spread the croutons over a baking sheet and bake for about 15 minutes, or until the croutons are golden, crisp, and fragrant. Set aside.

3   Make the soup: In a large pot, heat the olive oil over medium-high heat. Once the oil starts to shimmer, add the onion and garlic and cook until translucent, about 3 minutes. Add the cashews, thyme, salt, paprika, and turmeric and cook for another minute. Stir in the carrot and cauliflower along with 2 cups (480 ml) of water. Bring the mixture to a boil, reduce to a simmer, and cook for 10 to 15 minutes, or until the vegetables are soft. Season with the yeast and more salt, if needed.

4   Carefully transfer the mixture to a blender and puree until smooth. (If you have one, an immersion blender is great here.) Add a few tablespoons of water, if you'd like a thinner consistency. Transfer the soup back into the pot and cover to keep warm if not serving right away. Otherwise, ladle the soup into 4 bowls, top with the croutons, and drizzle with oil.

KELP NOODLE CHAP CHAE

Chap chae is a traditional Korean dish that is essentially noodles topped with loads of vegetables. Our variation ups the healing quotient by using kelp noodles, which you can find in the Asian section of most stores and which deliver all the mineralizing goodness of sea vegetables. They get topped with a healthy heap of stir-fried veggies like bok choy, mushrooms, spinach, and cabbage, and are drizzled with a toasted sesame and ginger sauce. Here's to plant medicine, one delicious meal at a time!

SERVES 4

FOR THE NOODLES

1 (12-ounce/340 g) package
  kelp noodles

1 tablespoon apple cider
  vinegar

1 teaspoon baking soda

½ cup (30 g) sun-dried
  tomatoes, soaked for
  30 minutes in boiling
  water, drained, and
  chopped

¼ cup (60 ml) tahini

2 tablespoons tamari soy sauce

1 tablespoon wildflower honey

1 tablespoon toasted sesame oil

2 teaspoons chopped fresh
  ginger

2 cloves garlic, peeled

1½ teaspoons mirin

1½ teaspoons brown rice
  vinegar

FOR THE SAUTÉED VEGETABLES

2 heads bok choy

1 tablespoon extra-virgin
  olive oil

4 cups (500 g) shiitake
  mushrooms, stems
  removed and sliced ¼-inch
  (6 mm) thick

8 cups (240 g) baby spinach

2 cups (200 g) sliced or
  shredded red cabbage

½ teaspoon Himalayan salt, or
  more to taste

FOR FINISHING

1 large carrot, thinly sliced into
  ribbons

4 scallions (white and light
  green parts), thinly sliced

2 tablespoons sesame seeds

RECIPE CONTINUES

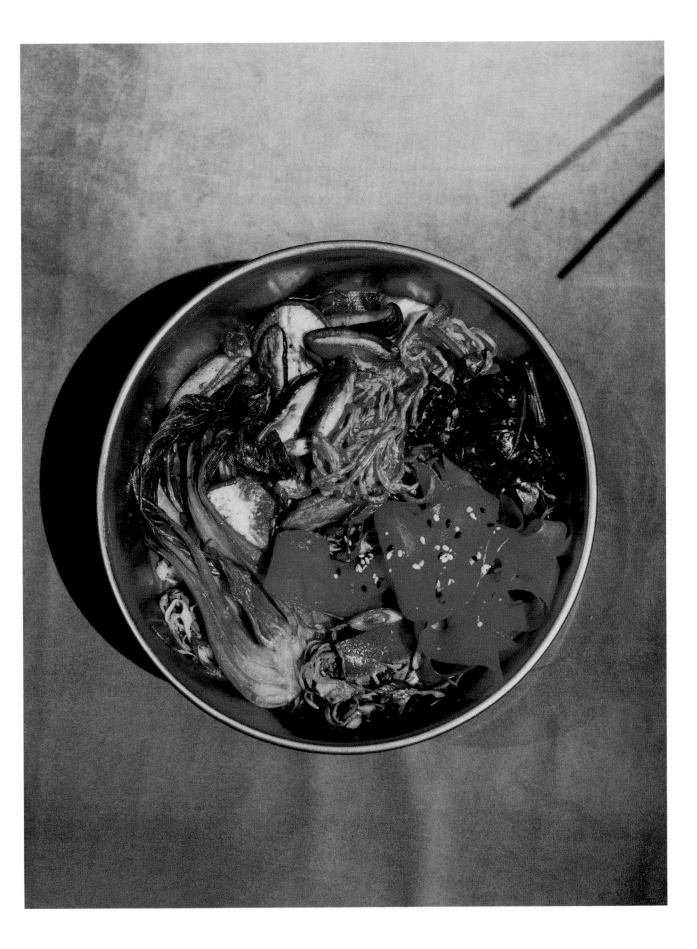

1   Make the noodles: In a large bowl, combine the kelp noodles, apple cider vinegar, and baking soda with enough warm water just to cover the noodles. Let the noodles soak for 30 minutes to make them nice and soft.

2   In a blender, combine all the remaining ingredients with ½ cup (120 ml) of water and blend until smooth. Add more water to loosen the consistency, if necessary; you want it to resemble a thick dressing. Set aside.

3   Make the vegetables: Trim the stem end of the bok choy and separate the leaves of each head.

4   In a large sauté pan, heat the oil over medium heat. When the oil begins to shimmer, add the mushrooms and sauté until softened and just beginning to brown, 2 to 3 minutes. Add the bok choy and cook for another 3 minutes to soften. Add the spinach, cabbage, and salt and continue to cook and stir the vegetables for 5 minutes, or until the cabbage has softened and the spinach has wilted. Taste and add salt, if desired.

5   Strain the noodles and rinse thoroughly, then spread them out over a clean dishtowel or paper towels. Pat the noodles dry with another layer of towels.

6   In a large bowl, combine the noodles with the carrots, scallions, and half of the sauce. Toss until evenly combined. Top with the cooked vegetables and toss with the remaining sauce. Sprinkle with the sesame seeds and serve.

MELON POKE BOWL
+ CITRUS PONZU AND COCONUT LENTILS

We summon this client favorite when we want to feel the island breezes in our hair. It's pulled straight from our menu and is our even lighter take on the Hawaiian cult hit, which usually includes raw fish. Ours, however, feature super-hydrating melon dipped in a citrus-soy marinade; handfuls of sesame-, hemp-, dulse-, and spicy kochukaro–speckled avocado; and is topped with a tuft of potent homemade pickled ginger. We serve it all over coconut milk–simmered lentils and welcome thoughts of sun-warmed beaches.

SERVES 4

FOR THE MELON POKE

½ cup (120 ml) tamari soy sauce

¼ cup (60 ml) fresh orange juice

¼ cup (60 ml) fresh lime juice

¼ cup (60 ml) fresh grapefruit juice

2 tablespoons mirin

4 cups (610 g) watermelon, diced into ½-inch (12 mm) cubes

3 cups (510 g) honeydew melon, diced into ½-inch (12 mm) cubes

FOR THE PICKLED GINGER

2 tablespoons beet kvass or beet juice

1 (3-inch/7.5 cm) knob fresh ginger, peeled and shaved thin with a mandoline or vegetable peeler (about ½ cup/50 g)

⅓ cup (75 ml) brown rice vinegar

2 tablespoons wildflower honey

FOR THE COCONUT LENTILS

1 cup (200 g) beluga or French lentils

1½ tablespoons coconut oil

2 tablespoons sliced shallots

¼ teaspoon Himalayan salt

½ cup (120 ml) coconut milk

FOR THE CRUSTED AVOCADO

1 teaspoon dulse

½ teaspoon hemp seeds

¼ teaspoon kochukaru

¼ teaspoon black sesame seeds

¼ teaspoon white sesame seeds

1 large avocado, pitted and diced

FOR FINISHING

12 cups (240 g) mizuna lettuce or arugula

1 cup (133 g) peeled and sliced English cucumbers

3 thinly sliced scallions (white and green parts)

2 thinly sliced radishes

2 thinly sliced watermelon radishes

RECIPE CONTINUES

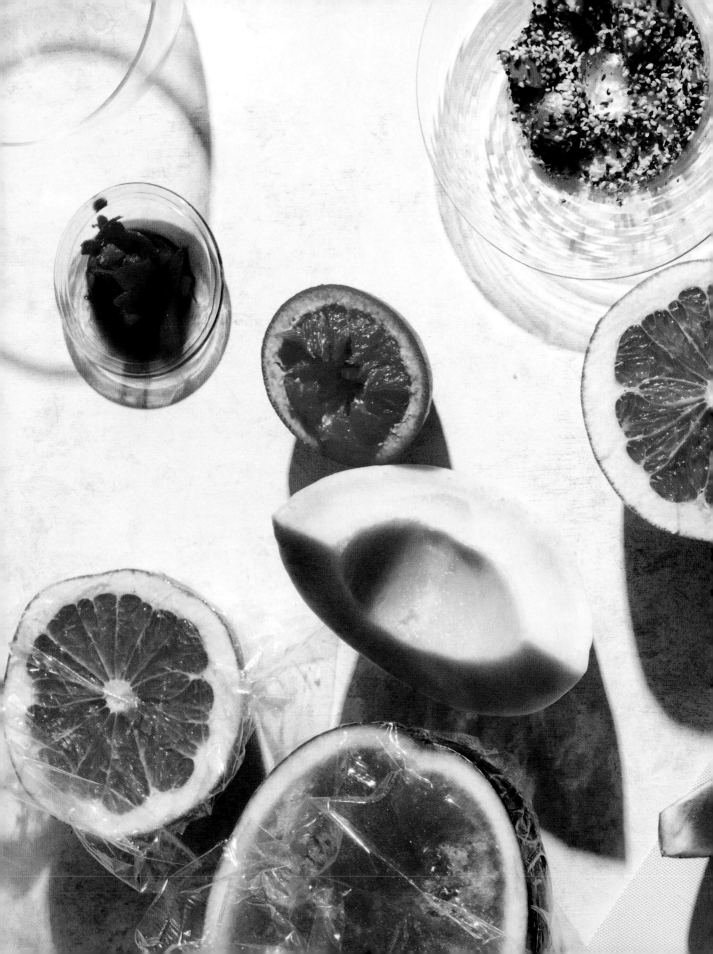

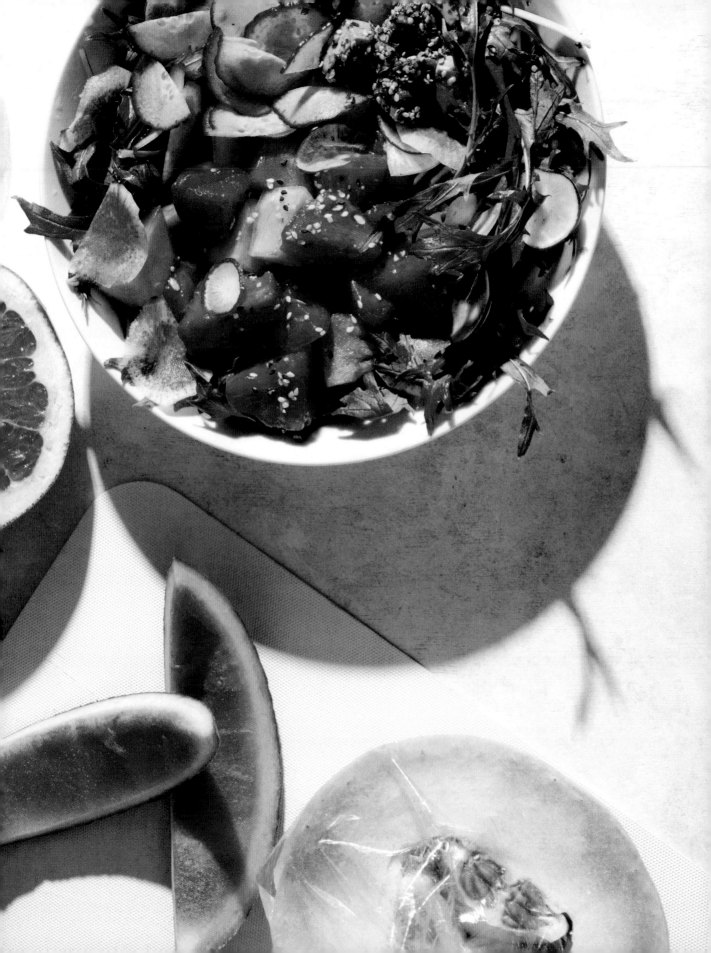

1   Make the melon poke: In a large bowl, make the citrus ponzu by whisking together the tamari, orange juice, lime juice, grapefruit juice, and mirin until combined. Gently toss the watermelon and honeydew in the ponzu to coat. Cover with plastic wrap and marinate in the fridge for at least 4 hours or overnight.

2   Make the pickled ginger: In a medium bowl, combine the kvass and the shaved ginger. Set aside.

3   In a small pot, bring the vinegar and honey to a boil over high heat, stirring until the honey dissolves. Remove the pot from the heat and pour the vinegar mixture over the ginger mixture. Allow to cool to room temperature and chill in the fridge for at least 1 hour or overnight.

4   Make the lentils: In a medium pot, combine the lentils with 4 cups (960 ml) of water and bring to a boil. Reduce to a simmer and cook partially covered for 20 to 30 minutes, or until the lentils are tender. Drain off any excess water.

5   In a large skillet, heat the oil over medium-high heat. When the oil shimmers, add the shallots and cook, stirring constantly, for 1 to 2 minutes, or until just starting to brown. Add the cooked lentils and salt and stir to combine. Stir in the milk, then remove the pot from the heat. Let the lentils cool to room temperature.

6   Make the crusted avocado: In a small bowl, stir together the dulse, hemp seeds, kochukaru, black sesame seeds, and white sesame seeds.

7   In a medium bowl, add the diced avocado and sprinkle about half of the seed mixture over the top. Toss very gently to combine, then add the remaining seed mixture and toss again until the avocado is evenly coated.

8   Assemble the bowl: Remove the melon from the marinade. Arrange the lettuce in a serving bowl and top with the lentils and melon poke, reserving the ponzu. Sprinkle the avocado, sliced cucumbers, scallions, and radishes over the top and garnish with the pickled ginger. Drizzle with the ponzu and serve.

ROASTED PEACH CHANA MASALA
+ COCONUT QUINOA AND MINT CHUTNEY

Chana masala, an Indian dish that features chickpeas simmered in a spiced tomato-based sauce, is alluringly complex in flavor but refreshingly simple to make at home. Our version has a few updated twists: Cinnamon-dusted peaches, turmeric, and coconut palm sugar for a sweet-spiced touch, and a drizzle of mint chutney infused with triphala, an herbal formula that's been used by Ayurvedic healers for two thousand years to soothe and strengthen the digestive system and stoke the metabolism.

SERVES 4 TO 6

FOR THE MINT CHUTNEY

2½ tablespoons extra-virgin olive oil

1 tablespoon fresh lemon juice

1 cup (25 g) fresh mint leaves

1 cup (50 g) packed fresh cilantro leaves

½ small serrano chile, seeded and chopped

1 teaspoon wildflower honey

¼ teaspoon triphala (1 capsule)

Himalayan salt

FOR THE ROASTED PEACHES

3 peaches, cut into ½-inch (12 mm) slices

1 tablespoon extra-virgin olive oil

1 teaspoon ground cinnamon

1 teaspoon ground turmeric

1 teaspoon coconut palm sugar

¼ teaspoon Himalayan salt

FOR THE QUINOA

⅔ cup (110 g) uncooked white quinoa

1½ cups (360 ml) coconut milk

½ teaspoon Himalayan salt

FOR THE CHANA MASALA

2 tablespoons extra-virgin olive oil

1 medium onion, chopped

¼ cup (60 ml) tomato paste

4 cloves garlic, minced

1 (1-inch/2.5 cm) knob fresh ginger, peeled and minced or grated

1 teaspoon ground coriander

2 teaspoons ground cumin

1½ teaspoons garam masala

1 teaspoon ground turmeric

1 teaspoon coconut palm sugar

1 teaspoon Himalayan salt, or more to taste

½ teaspoon freshly ground black pepper

2 (14-ounce/400 g) cans chickpeas, rinsed and drained

1 (14-ounce/400 g) can crushed tomatoes

2 large carrots, sliced into ¼-inch (6 mm) rounds

1½ tablespoons maple syrup

¾ cup (180 ml) Orgasmic Coconut Yogurt (page 62) or store-bought

1 lime

FOR FINISHING

2 tablespoons hemp seeds, for garnish

Fresh mint (optional)

Sautéed Daily Greens (page 33; optional)

DINNER

RECIPE CONTINUES

1   Make the chutney: In a blender or food processor, combine all the ingredients and blend until smooth. You may need to add a small amount of water to help loosen the mixture. Season with salt to taste and set aside.

2   Make the roasted peaches: Preheat the oven to 350°F (175°C). Line a baking sheet with parchment paper and set aside.

3   In a medium bowl, toss the peaches with the oil, cinnamon, turmeric, sugar, and salt to evenly coat. Arrange the peaches in a single layer on the baking sheet and roast for 20 minutes, or until the peaches are soft yet still hold their shape. Set aside.

4   Make the quinoa: In a medium pot, bring the quinoa and milk to a boil over medium heat, then reduce the heat to low, cover, and simmer for 15 minutes, or until the quinoa is tender. Remove from the heat and allow to cool for 5 minutes before fluffing with a fork. Cover and set aside.

5   Make the chana masala: In a large skillet, heat the olive oil over medium-high heat. Add the onion and sauté until just turning translucent, about 2 minutes. Stir in the tomato paste, garlic, ginger, coriander, cumin, 1 teaspoon of the garam masala, turmeric, sugar, salt, and pepper. Continue stirring as the spices toast and the mixture becomes fragrant, about 1 minute. Stir in the chickpeas, tomatoes, carrots, and maple syrup with ½ cup (120 ml) of water. Bring the mixture to a simmer, reduce the heat to low, and cook for 15 minutes, or until the carrots are tender and the mixture is thickened. Stir in the remaining ½ teaspoon of garam masala, the yogurt, and a squeeze of lime to taste. Gently simmer for 10 more minutes. Taste and add more salt, if desired.

6   To assemble: Spread the quinoa over a platter or wide serving bowl. Top with the chickpea mixture, followed by the peaches. Drizzle the mint chutney over the top and garnish with hemp seeds and mint, if desired. We recommend a side of simply sautéed Daily Greens.

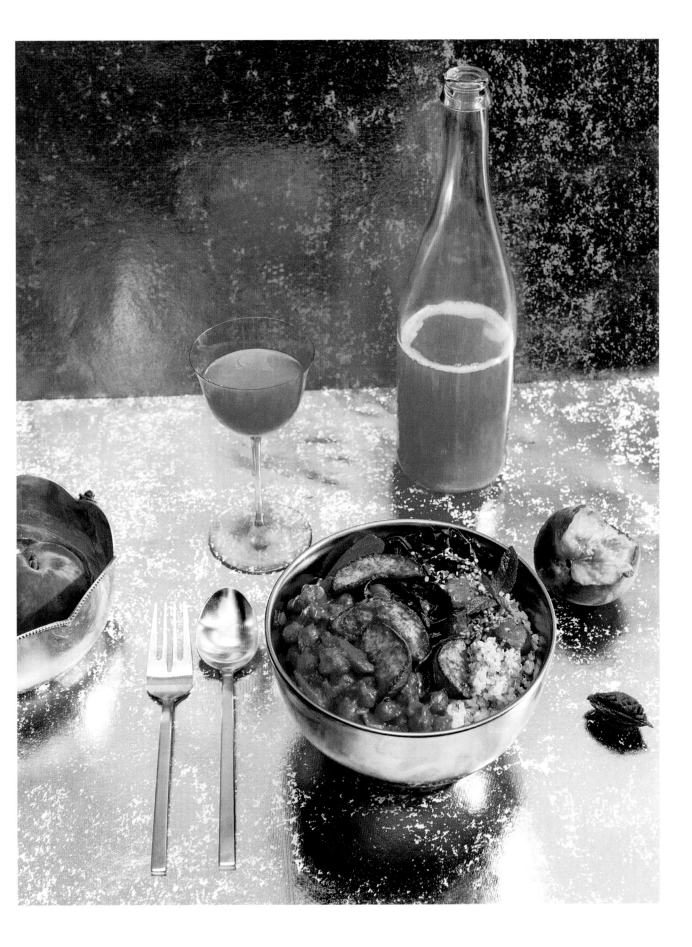

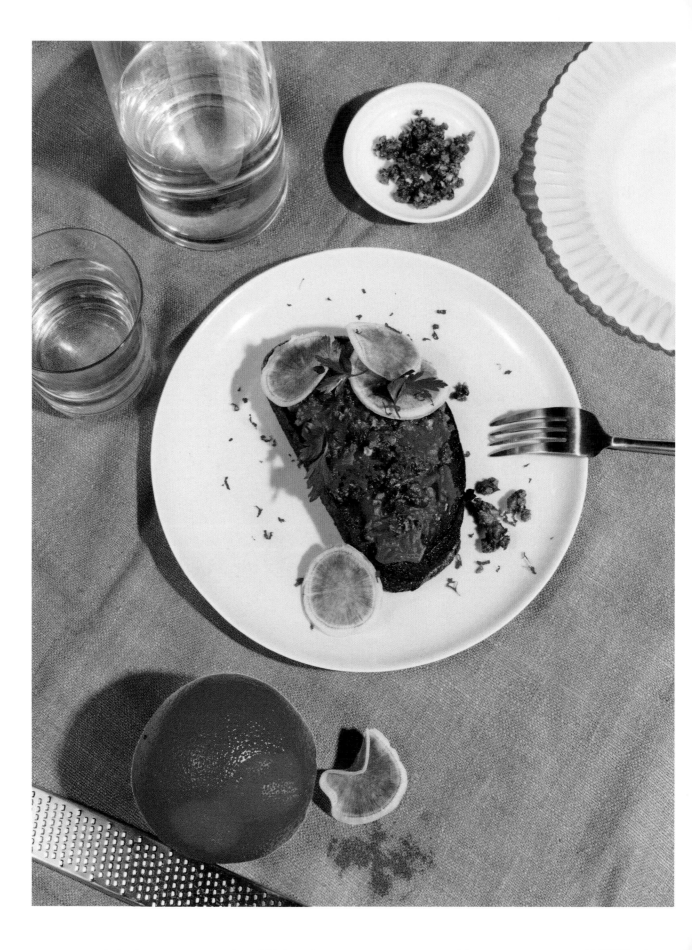

SWEET POTATO TARTINES WITH WALNUT GREMOLATA

FOR THE SWEET POTATOES

1 large sweet potato, peeled and cut into 1-inch (2.5 cm) cubes

1 tablespoon extra-virgin olive oil

¼ teaspoon Himalayan salt, or more to taste

1 teaspoon maple syrup

FOR THE WALNUT GREMOLATA

½ cup (50 g) walnuts

8 sprigs fresh cilantro, stems discarded

4 sprigs fresh parsley, stems discarded, plus more for garnish

1 tablespoon extra-virgin olive oil

2 cloves garlic

Zest and juice of 1 lemon

Zest of 1 orange

¼ teaspoon Himalayan salt

FOR FINISHING

2 slices Sakara Seed Bread (page 187) or gluten-free bread

1 watermelon radish, thinly sliced

We don't think we'll ever get sick of avocado toast, but sometimes we could use a little something to change it up. Our suggestion? Sweet potato toast! Or *tartines*, if you're feeling fancy—and we most certainly are. We roast the orange vitamin A–filled beauties to caramelized perfection, whip them with a bit of salt and maple syrup, and top off the mash with a dollop of gremolata, a sunny blend of walnuts, fresh herbs, and citrus. Enjoy with Daily Greens (page 33) on the side—or piled on your tartines! We like pairing this with wilted spinach lightly dressed with olive oil and lemon juice.

1   Make the sweet potatoes: Preheat the oven to 375°F (190°C).

2   On a baking sheet, toss the potatoes with the oil and salt. Arrange them in a single layer and roast for 15 to 20 minutes, or until very soft. Transfer the potatoes to a medium bowl and mash with a fork. Stir in the maple syrup. Taste and add a pinch of salt, if desired. Set aside.

3   Make the gremolata: In a dry pan, toast the walnuts over medium-low heat until they're fragrant, about 5 minutes. Allow the walnuts to cool slightly, then add them to a food processor with the cilantro, parsley, oil, garlic, lemon zest and juice, orange zest, and salt. Pulse until the mixture comes together but is still crumbly.

4   Assemble the toast: Lightly toast the bread in a toaster or in the oven for 3 to 5 minutes. Heap the warm toast with the mashed sweet potatoes, dollop with the gremolata, and top with radish slices.

DINNER

LENTIL SOUP WITH COCONUT YOGURT

1 tablespoon extra-virgin
olive oil

1 medium carrot, sliced into
thin rounds

2 cups (215 g) cauliflower
florets

½ small yellow onion, finely
diced

2 cloves garlic, thinly sliced

1 tablespoon minced fresh
ginger

¾ cup (150 g) red lentils

3 tablespoons tomato paste

2 teaspoons ground cumin

1 teaspoon chili powder

Juice of 1 orange

¼ teaspoon Himalayan salt, or
more to taste

Freshly ground black pepper

2 tablespoons Orgasmic
Coconut Yogurt (page 62)
or store-bought, plus more
for serving

2 sprigs fresh mint, leaves
picked and torn

There's something about a pot of soup on a crisp day that sets the heart free. This soothing hug of a stew blends lentils' hearty nourishing power with cauliflower's natural body, with a hint of warmth and smokiness from chili powder and cumin, and a drizzle of coconut yogurt for a creamy, tangy finish. We love capping it off with a sprig of fresh mint, as a gentle reminder that greener days are ahead.

In a medium pot, heat the oil over medium heat. Add the carrot and sauté for 3 minutes, just to sweat. Add the cauliflower, onion, garlic, and ginger and continue to sauté, stirring occasionally, until the cauliflower begins to soften, about 5 minutes. If the bottom of the pan starts to look dry, add 1 tablespoon of water. Add the lentils, tomato paste, spices, and orange juice and cook for 2 minutes to lightly brown the tomato paste and toast the spices. Stir in 4 cups (960 ml) of water along with the salt and a few cracks of black pepper. Bring the soup to a boil, reduce the heat to low, cover, and simmer for 20 minutes, or until the lentils are tender. Remove from the heat, taste and add salt, if necessary, and fold in the coconut yogurt. Ladle the soup into bowls and garnish with a dollop of yogurt and the mint leaves.

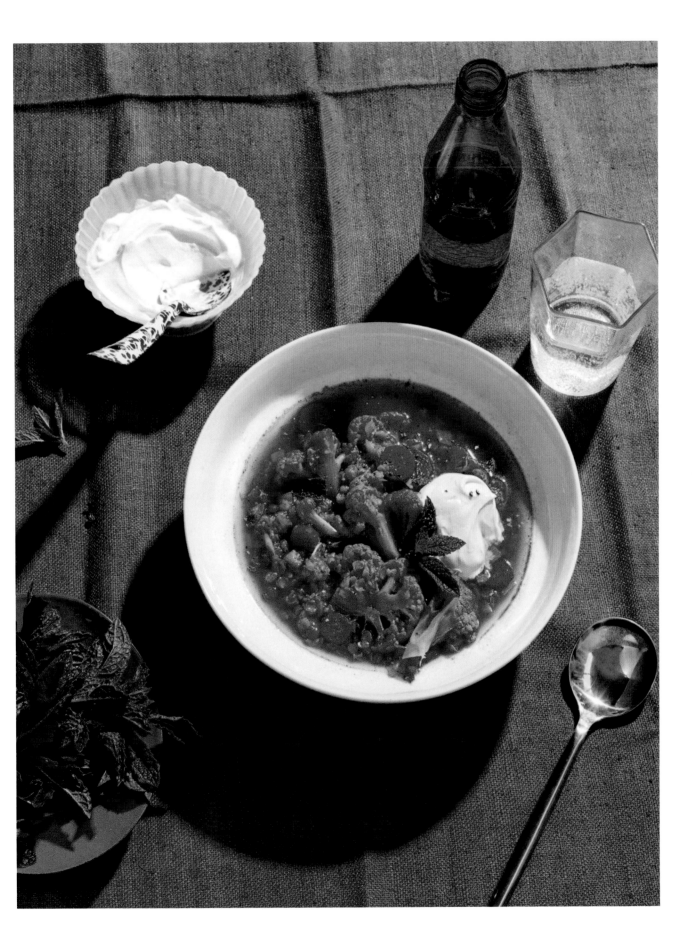

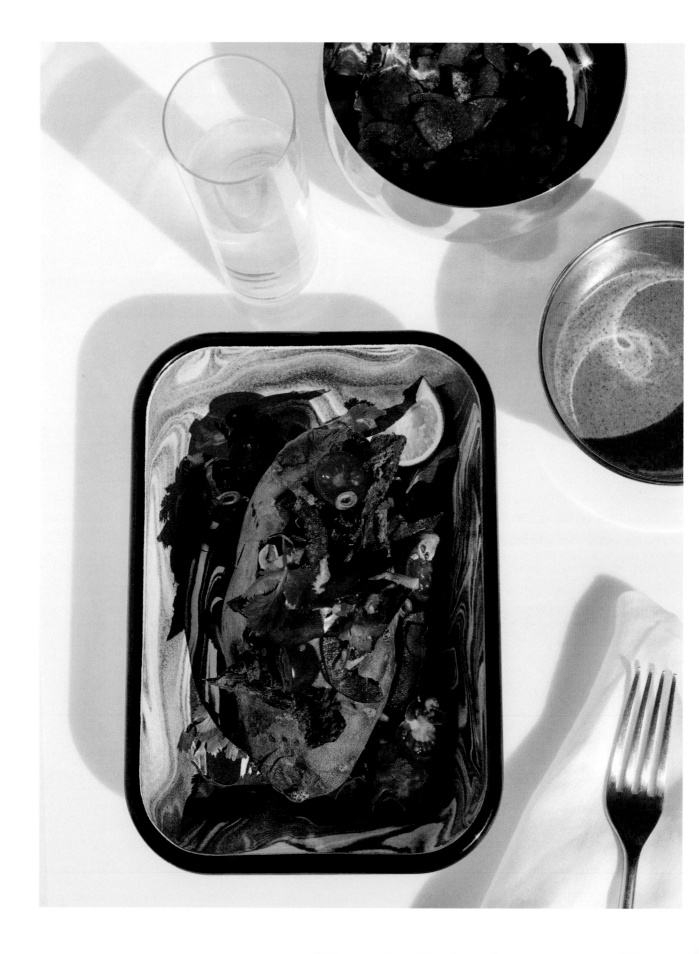

LOADED SWEET POTATOES

SERVES 4

FOR THE SWEET POTATOES

4 large purple sweet potatoes
  (go with medium if you're
  using an orange variety)

FOR THE COCONUT "BACON"

1 cup (85 g) coconut flakes

2 teaspoons tamari soy sauce

½ teaspoon wildflower honey

¼ teaspoon ground paprika

FOR THE "SOUR CREAM"

½ cup (80 g) hemp seeds

2 tablespoons fresh lemon juice

2 tablespoons nutritional yeast

½ teaspoon Himalayan salt, or
  more to taste

2 tablespoons chopped chives

FOR FINISHING

1 cup (170 g) cooked or canned
  black beans, rinsed and
  drained

½ cup (75 g) cherry tomatoes,
  halved

½ cup (25 g) chopped fresh
  cilantro

4 scallions (white and green
  parts), thinly sliced

1 lime, sliced into wedges

What is more tempting than a steaming hot potato stuffed with sour cream and bacon bits? Of course, our version showcases a velvety hemp seed "sour cream" and baked coconut "bacon" sprinkled over a purple Japanese sweet potato (which is similar in sweetness to its orange relatives, and just as beneficial), but the effect is the same: abundance for the body and the soul.

1 Make the sweet potatoes: Preheat the oven to 400°F (205°C).

2 Line a rimmed baking sheet with parchment paper or foil. Arrange the potatoes on the baking sheet and pierce them all over with a fork. Roast for 40 to 50 minutes, or until a small knife slides right through the center. Set aside and cover with foil or a clean towel to keep the potatoes warm. Keep the oven on.

3 Make the coconut "bacon": In a medium bowl, combine all the ingredients. Evenly scatter the mixture over a baking sheet lined with parchment paper and bake for 3 to 5 minutes, or until golden brown. Set aside.

4 Make the "sour cream": In a blender, combine the hemp seeds, lemon juice, yeast, and salt with ¼ cup (60 ml) of water and blend until smooth. Add more water if you'd like a looser consistency, and add more salt to taste. Fold in the chives.

5 Assemble the loaded potatoes: Slice each sweet potato lengthwise, taking care not to cut them completely in half. Open the potatoes as you would a book and use a spoon to gently press down the potato meat into the skin, making room for all the toppings. Top with the beans and tomatoes. Sprinkle each potato with the coconut "bacon," scallions, and, of course, a dollop of "sour cream." Finish with a squeeze of lime.

SAKARA PAD THAI

Before pad thai was a takeout staple, it was a dish that helped bring an entire country to better health. In the late 1930s, in an effort to encourage the people of Thailand to enjoy inexpensive but nutrient-dense meals, the prime minister urged them to make pad thai—which up until then was a traditionally Chinese dish. With its inexpensive and filling rice noodles, ample vegetables, and simple but fortifying proteins all tossed in a bright, spicy chili sauce, it was the perfect solution. Even though the modern restaurant version of this dish isn't exactly healthful, at its heart pad thai is as nourishing as it is flavorful. Our recipe features high-quality, healing ingredients like broccoli, mushrooms, carrots, spinach, and tempeh, plus a chili-lime sauce for a dish that's truly noble in its humility.

SERVES 4

FOR THE STIR-FRIED VEGETABLES

2 tablespoons sesame oil

1 large head broccoli, chopped into bite-size florets

1 cup (125 g) shiitake mushrooms, stemmed and sliced into ¼-inch (6 mm) slices

1 (8-ounce/225 g) package unflavored tempeh, cut into ½-inch (12 mm) pieces

2 large carrots, thinly sliced into ribbons

4 cups (120 g) packed spinach

1½ tablespoons tamari soy sauce

1 teaspoon Himalayan salt

FOR THE SAUCE

1 teaspoon red pepper flakes

Juice of 2 limes

2 tablespoons sesame oil

2 tablespoons sunflower oil

¼ cup (60 ml) tamari soy sauce

2½ tablespoons wildflower honey

FOR FINISHING

1 (8-ounce/225 g) package pad thai rice noodles

4 scallions (white and green parts), thinly sliced on the bias

8 sprigs fresh cilantro, leaves roughly chopped

¼ cup (35 g) almonds, roughly chopped

1 lime, sliced into wedges

Red pepper flakes or your favorite sriracha (optional)

RECIPE CONTINUES

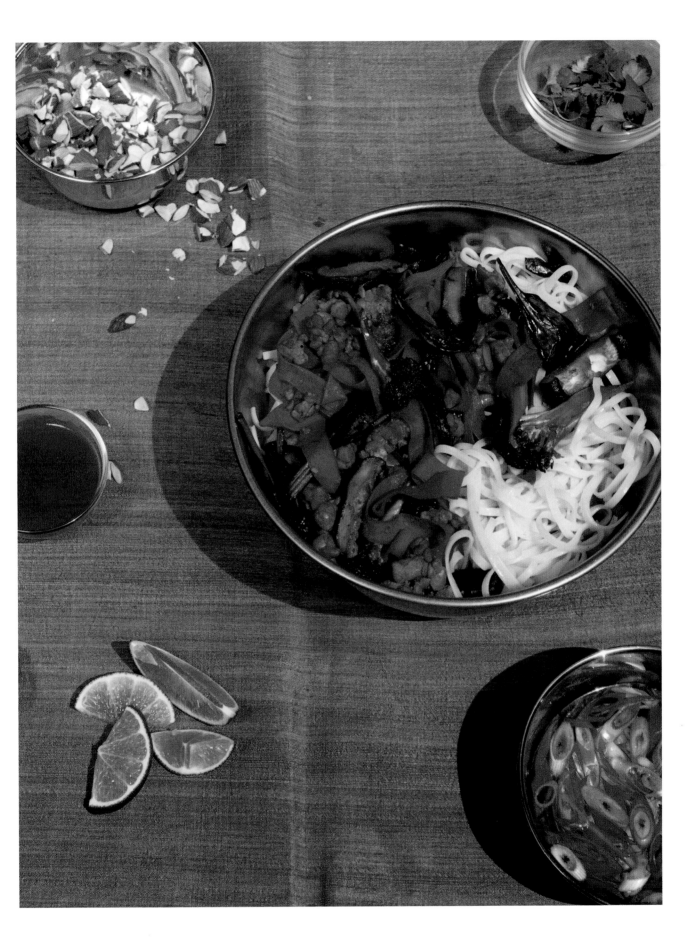

1   Make the vegetables: In a large skillet, heat the oil over medium heat. When the oil starts to shimmer, add the broccoli, mushrooms, and tempeh and cover. Cook for 15 minutes, stirring occasionally, or until the broccoli is tender. Add the carrots, spinach, tamari, and salt. Toss to combine and cook while stirring for 2 to 3 minutes, or until the spinach is just wilted. Set aside.

2   Make the sauce: In a medium bowl, whisk together all the ingredients with ¼ cup (60 ml) of water. Set aside.

3   Assemble the pad thai: Fill a large pot with water and bring to a boil. Cook the noodles according to the package instructions and drain.

4   In a large bowl, toss the stir-fried vegetables and tempeh with half of the sauce, along with the scallions and cilantro.

5   In another large bowl, dress the noodles with the remaining sauce. Top with the vegetables and sprinkle with the almonds. Serve with lime wedges and red pepper flakes or sriracha, if desired.

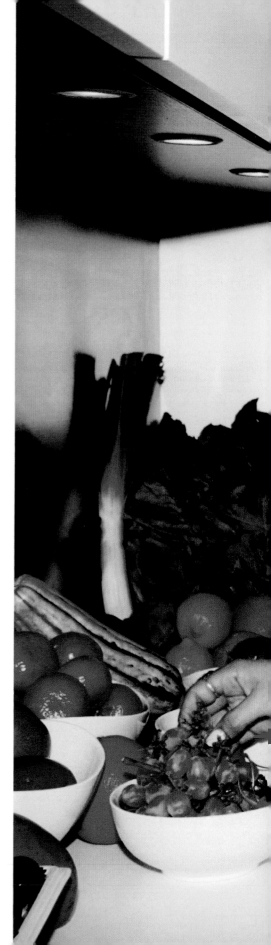

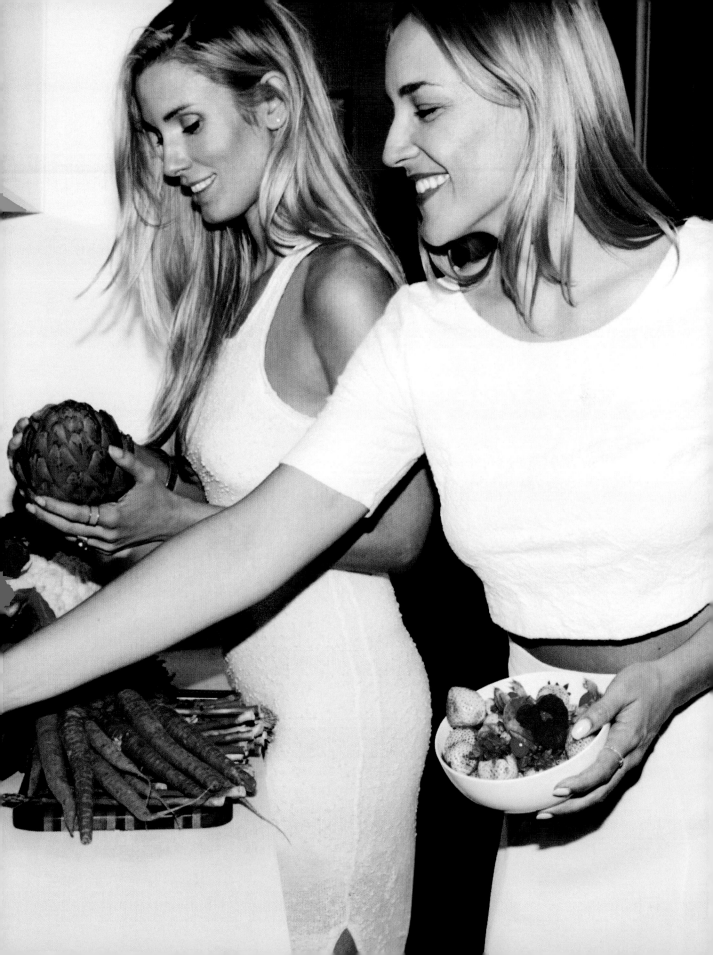

SAKARA "LOUIE"

Get a bite of West Coast vibes with this creamy, refreshing salad. It hits all the same tasty notes as a classic seafood Louie, with cleverly used plant-based ingredients providing the satisfying texture and substance (while keeping it pleasantly light and fresh). Our recipe calls for tossing potassium-rich, hydrating hearts of palm; crisp, cleansing red bell pepper; and immunity-supporting, glow-bestowing carrots with a luxurious cashew-and-fresh-herb dressing. What you get is a satisfying salad that's equally at home in a sandwich or scooped atop a bed of greens. While the true origins of the classic Louie are contested, this version springs from our mission to create plant-based dishes that require no compromise, leaving you feeling perfectly fulfilled in body and spirit.

SERVES 4
███

FOR THE CASHEW-HERB DRESSING

¼ cup (30 g) cashews, soaked overnight

3 fresh chives, roughly chopped

Juice of 1 lemon

1 tablespoon packed fresh parsley leaves

1 tablespoon packed fresh dill fronds

1 teaspoon apple cider vinegar

¼ teaspoon Himalayan salt, or more to taste

FOR THE LOUIE MIX

1 (14-ounce/400 g) can hearts of palm, drained and finely diced

1 red bell pepper, finely diced

1 small carrot, grated

1 stalk of celery, finely diced

1 medium shallot, minced

Himalayan salt and freshly ground black pepper

FOR THE SALAD

8 cups (240 g) mixed greens

2 avocados, pitted and sliced

1 cup (150 g) cherry tomatoes, quartered

½ cucumber, sliced into thin ribbons

2 tablespoons hemp seeds

Juice of ½ lemon

1 tablespoon extra-virgin olive oil

Himalayan salt

FOR FINISHING

8 pieces Sakara Seed Bread (page 187) or gluten-free bread (optional)

Sliced tomatoes

Sliced red onions

Pickles

RECIPE CONTINUES

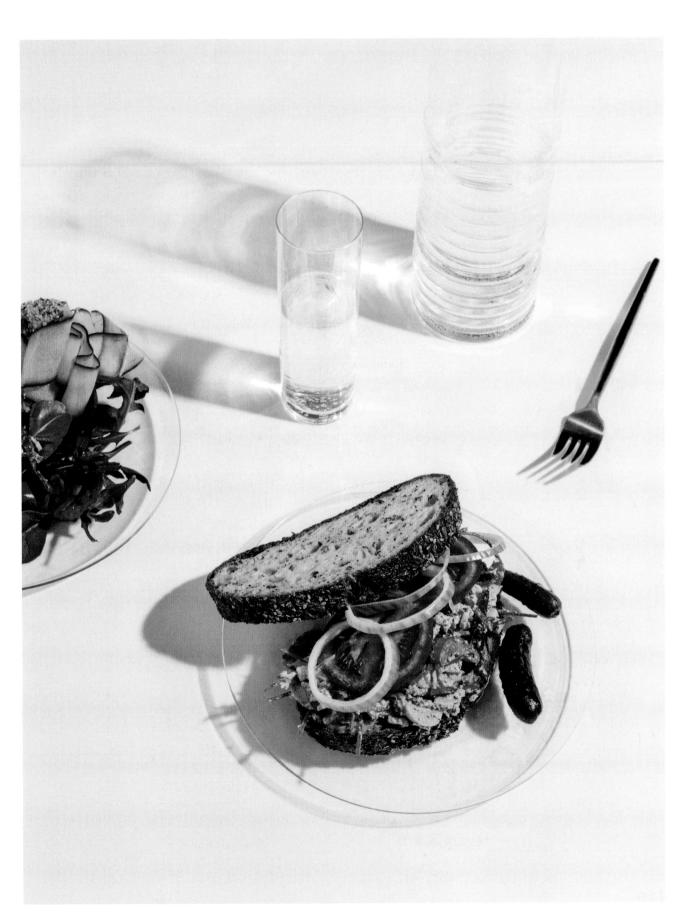

1   Make the dressing: In a blender, puree all the ingredients with 2 tablespoons of water until smooth and creamy. Season with more salt, if desired.

2   Make the Louie mix: In a medium bowl, toss all the ingredients with the dressing. Season with a pinch of salt and a few cracks of pepper.

3   Make the salad: In a large bowl, combine the greens with the avocados, tomatoes, cucumber, and hemp seeds. Add the lemon juice, oil, and a pinch of salt. Toss to evenly coat.

4   Assemble: Either scoop the Louie mixture on top of the greens or divide the mixture among 4 slices of bread, top with the sliced tomatoes and onions, and finish with another piece of bread. Enjoy the salad on the sandwich or on the side. We like to serve it up with some pickles.

GARLIC

USED IN *traditional healing* FOR *centuries*

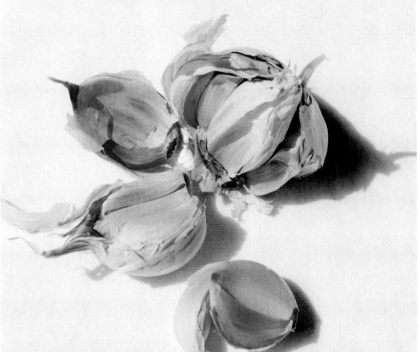

GARLIC IS A RUTHLESS ASSASSIN OF COLDS AND INFECTIONS.

When we were just beginning to experiment with food as medicine, one of our first trials was an intense garlic cleanse in which we ate huge amounts of this pungent allium with the hope of killing off candida and flushing out toxins. It may not have been awesome for our breath, but we can see why this remedy has been used in traditional healing for centuries. As one of the most potent natural antimicrobials, antivirals, and antifungals, garlic (and one of its chemical compounds called allicin) is a ruthless assassin of illness-causing microorganisms. Enjoying garlic (especially raw) on a regular basis can help prevent colds and infections. It's also great for regulating blood sugar levels, reducing LDL cholesterol and blood pressure, increasing circulation, and preventing and reversing heart disease. A couple insider tips: Garlic can be hard on your stomach when eaten by itself, so we recommend keeping it mixed into meals and also chewing on a little mint before hanging out with your friends . . .

DINNER

141

CLASSIC STIR-FRY

SERVES 4

FOR THE PICKLED CHILES

2 serrano chiles, seeded and
 thinly sliced

¼ cup (60 ml) brown rice
 vinegar

2 tablespoons maple syrup

FOR THE STIR-FRY

¼ cup (60 ml) almond butter

4 cloves garlic, minced

1 tablespoon tamari soy sauce

Zest and juice of 2 limes

3 tablespoons sunflower oil

1 small red onion, sliced

1 large head broccoli, chopped
 into bite-size florets

½ small head purple cabbage,
 shredded (about 2 cups/
 200 g)

2 tablespoons minced or grated
 fresh ginger

3 cups (555 g) cooked quinoa

2 large carrots, grated

4 cups (120 g) spinach

Himalayan salt

1 small bunch fresh cilantro,
 leaves roughly chopped

4 scallions (white and green
 parts), thinly sliced

This is one of our favorite dishes to make because, in addition to naturally cleansing quinoa, broccoli, spinach, and cabbage, we've added a generous dose of one of our other favorite body-wide scrubbers: cilantro. The chemical compounds of this perfumed leafy green bind to heavy metals and other toxins; loosen them from your tissues, blood, and organs; and dispose of them properly. The oils from cilantro also work wonders on the digestive tract, triggering the production of digestive enzymes that help your body break food down and absorb more of its nutrients.

1   Make the pickled chiles: In a small pot, bring the chiles, vinegar, and maple syrup to a boil. Remove from the heat and let the chiles sit for at least 5 minutes or overnight. Store the pickled chiles in the fridge in their pickling liquid for up to 1 month.

2   Make the stir-fry: In a medium bowl, whisk together the almond butter, garlic, tamari, lime zest and juice, and ¼ cup (60 ml) of water.

3   In a large skillet, heat 2 tablespoons of the oil over high heat. Sauté the onion until just soft, about 1 minute. Add the broccoli to the pan in an even layer and let it sear, without stirring, for 2 minutes. Give the mixture a toss and continue cooking for another 5 minutes, stirring occasionally to avoid burning (though some charring is okay!). Add the remaining 1 tablespoon of oil, along with the cabbage and ginger. Cook until just tender, while stirring, about 3 minutes. Add the quinoa and cook for 2 minutes to lightly toast it, then stir in the almond butter mixture. Fold in the grated carrots and spinach and cook, while stirring, until the spinach has just wilted, about 2 minutes. Remove the pan from the heat, taste, and season with salt, if desired. Divide the stir-fry among 4 bowls and sprinkle with the cilantro, scallions, and pickled chiles strained from their liquid.

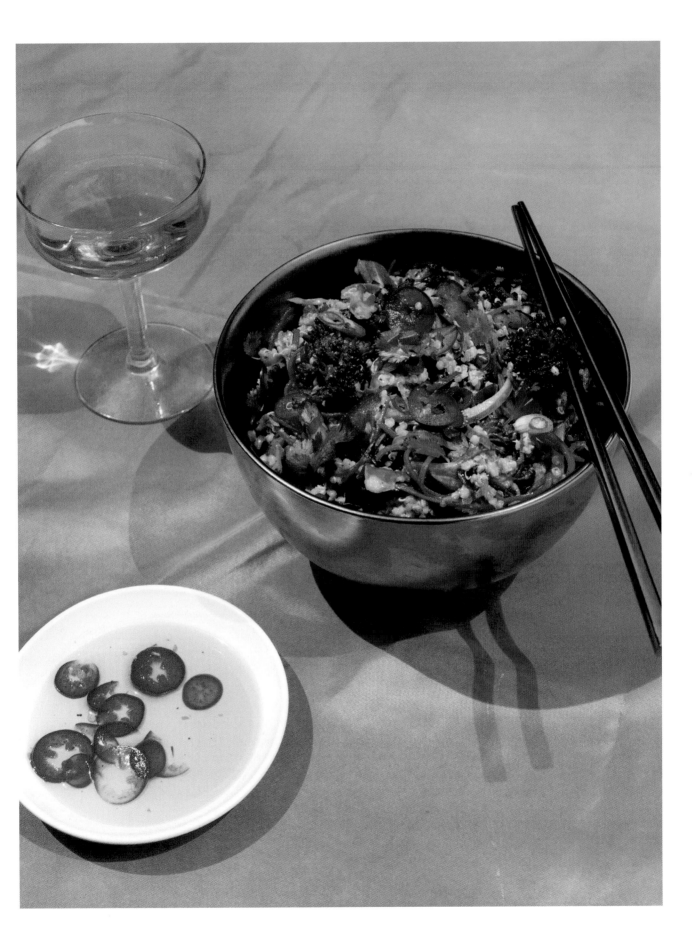

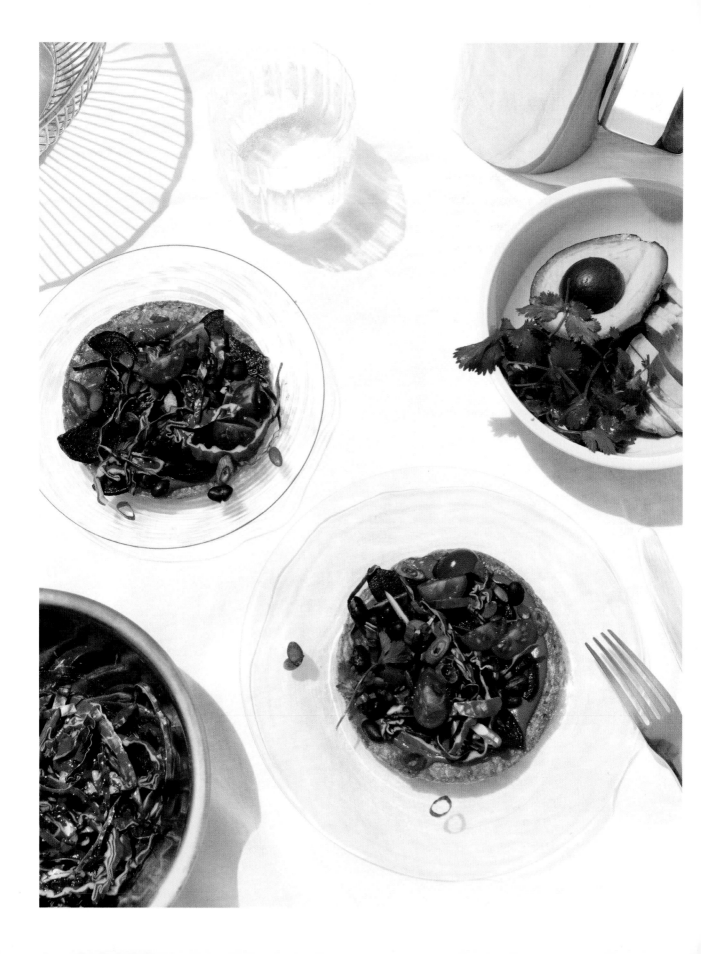

BEET TOSTADAS

We've delivered more than one million meals to clients all across the country and found that not everybody loves beets. So we challenged ourselves to come up with a dish to help those of you non-beet eaters join in the fun—there's no reason you should have to miss out on all those amazing detoxifying, blood-cleansing, endurance-boosting benefits! For this take on the classic taco truck offering, we pile up a crispy tortilla with a slather of "cheese" sauce, cumin-spiced roasted beets, and a raw veggie salad tossed with a bright chive vinaigrette. It's satisfying in all the right smoky, saucy ways, so we say: Give beets a chance!

SERVES 4

FOR THE ROASTED BEETS

1 large or 3 small beets, scrubbed and sliced into thin half-moons

½ teaspoon Himalayan salt

½ teaspoon ground cumin

1 tablespoon extra-virgin olive oil

1 tablespoon apple cider vinegar

FOR THE "CHEESE" SAUCE

1 cup (140 g) store-bought roasted red peppers, drained

½ cup (120 ml) tahini

Juice of ½ lemon

½ teaspoon ground cumin

½ teaspoon chili powder

¼ teaspoon smoked paprika

Himalayan salt, or more to taste

FOR THE CHIVE VINAIGRETTE

2 tablespoons finely chopped chives

¼ cup (60 ml) apple cider vinegar

¼ cup (60 ml) extra-virgin olive oil

Juice of ½ lemon

Himalayan salt

FOR FINISHING

2 heads Bibb lettuce

½ small head purple cabbage, shredded (about 2 cups/ 200 g)

1 cup (150 g) cherry tomatoes, quartered

1 cup (170 g) cooked or canned black beans, rinsed and drained

4 large or 8 small gluten-free tortillas

1 tablespoon extra-virgin olive oil

2 avocados, pitted and sliced

¼ cup (25 g) thinly sliced scallions (white and green parts)

2 tablespoons roughly chopped cilantro leaves

2 tablespoons pumpkin seeds

RECIPE CONTINUES

1　Make the beets: Preheat the oven to 450°F (230°C).

2　In a medium bowl, toss the beets with the salt, cumin, oil, and vinegar. Arrange the beets on a baking sheet and roast until soft and tender, about 20 minutes. Set aside to cool slightly.

3　Make the "cheese" sauce: In a blender or food processor, combine all the ingredients plus a pinch of salt and blend until smooth and creamy. Add 1 tablespoon of water to loosen, if necessary. Taste and season with more salt, if desired. Set aside.

4　Make the vinaigrette: In a medium bowl or a jar, combine all the ingredients with a pinch of salt and whisk or shake to blend well. Set aside.

5　Assemble the tostadas: In a large bowl, combine the lettuce, cabbage, tomatoes, and beans. Drizzle with just enough dressing to coat and toss. Save any leftover dressing in the fridge for up to 5 days.

6　In a small pot, heat the "cheese" sauce until just warm. Cover and set aside.

7　Heat a large sauté pan over medium-high heat. Lightly brush each tortilla with the oil and toast until crispy on both sides, about 1 minute per side.

8　Lay each crisped tortilla on a plate. Top with a healthy spread of "cheese" sauce, a layer of beets, and a mound of salad on top. Garnish with the avocados, scallions, cilantro, and pumpkin seeds. You can go for it and eat it with your hands, or feel free to use a knife and fork salad-style—we won't judge either way!

SPINACH-ARTICHOKE VELVET SOUP

3 tablespoons extra-virgin
   olive oil

1 medium yellow onion,
   roughly chopped

3 cloves garlic, roughly
   chopped

1 teaspoon Himalayan salt,
   or more to taste

1 large head cauliflower,
   trimmed and roughly
   chopped

4 cups (960 ml) unsweetened
   nut milk

1 (14-ounce/400 g) can
   artichoke hearts, drained
   and roughly chopped

1½ teaspoons nutritional yeast

1 cup (30 g) spinach

1 lemon

Microgreens, for garnish

Did you know that artichokes are actually part of the thistle family? And that this magical flower-vegetable has more antioxidants than almost every other vegetable? That's why we had to include it in one of our favorite creamy soups, which blends sulfur-rich cauliflower with leafy green spinach to create a soup that tastes like a healthy artichoke-spinach dip. We love pairing it with Daily Greens (page 33), such as simple wilted spinach with a squeeze of lemon juice and a drizzle of fruity extra-virgin olive oil.

1   In a large pot, heat 1 tablespoon of the olive oil over medium-high heat until it shimmers. Add the onion, garlic, and ¼ teaspoon of the salt. Sauté the mixture for 2 to 3 minutes, stirring occasionally, until the onion softens. Toss in the cauliflower with another ¼ teaspoon of the salt and sauté for another 5 minutes. If the bottom of the pot starts to look dry, add 1 tablespoon of water. Stir in the milk, artichokes, yeast, and the remaining ½ teaspoon of salt and bring the mixture to a simmer. Cover and reduce the heat to low. Cook until the cauliflower is soft, about 10 minutes. Stir in the spinach until just wilted, about 2 minutes, and remove the pot from the heat.

2   Carefully ladle the cooked soup into a blender and puree until smooth. You may need to work in batches. Return the soup to the pot and finish with a squeeze of lemon. Stir, taste, and season with more lemon and salt, if necessary. Garnish with microgreens and enjoy hot.

DINNER

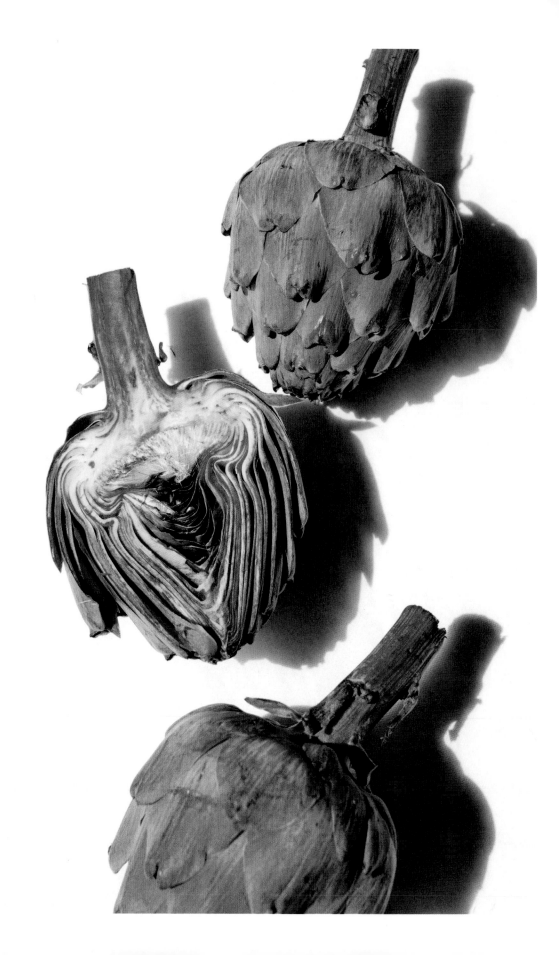

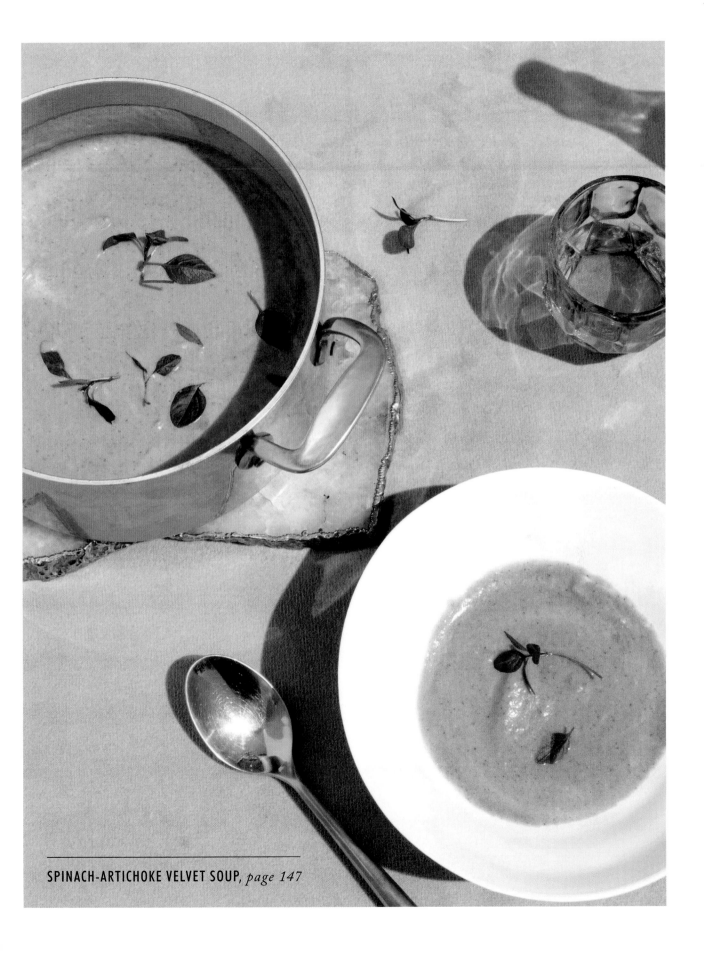

SPINACH-ARTICHOKE VELVET SOUP, *page 147*

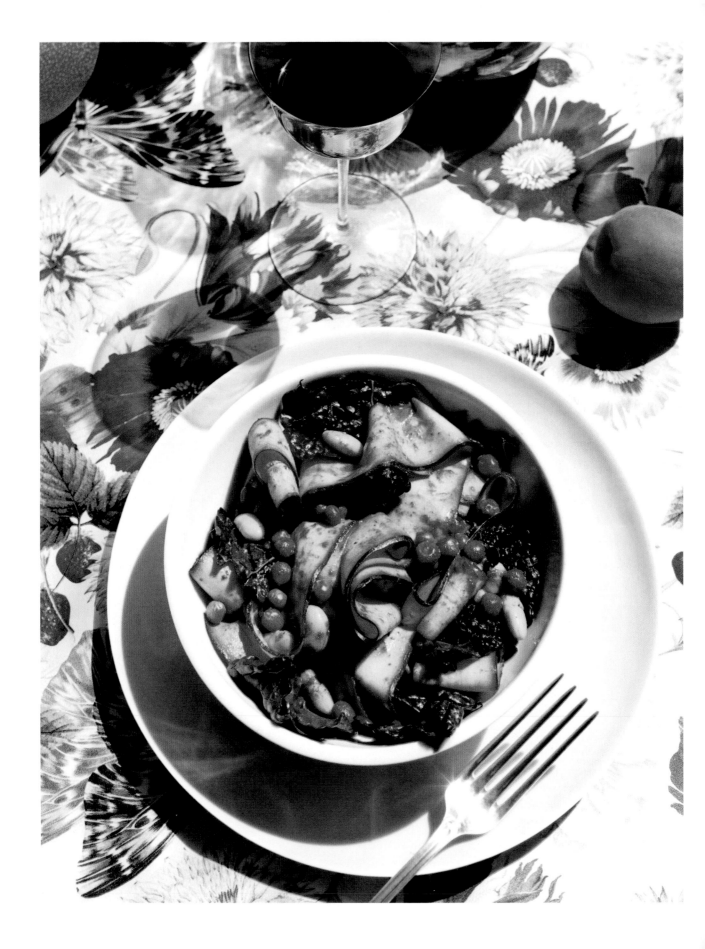

ZUCCHINI PESTO

SERVES 2

FOR THE HERB PISTOU

1 cup (30 g) baby spinach

4 sprigs fresh basil, leaves picked

2 sprigs fresh mint, leaves picked

2 sprigs fresh parsley, leaves picked

Zest and juice of 1 lemon

3 tablespoons extra-virgin olive oil

½ tablespoon white miso

1 clove garlic, roughly chopped

¼ teaspoon Himalayan salt, or more to taste

FOR THE PASTA

2 cups (42 g) roughly chopped kale

1 teaspoon extra-virgin olive oil

Himalayan salt

1 large zucchini, cut into ¼ by ¼-inch (6 by 6 mm) strips or spiralized into noodles, or 2 cups (240 g) store-bought zucchini noodles

½ cup (90 g) canned gigante or cannellini beans, strained and rinsed

½ cup (55 g) frozen peas, defrosted (or fresh, shelled peas if they are in season)

1 teaspoon fresh lemon juice

Fresh spring green is what it's all about for this play on pasta. We channeled the South of France and its lavender-scented breezes for inspiration, layering a bed of vitamin- and fiber-rich, ultrahydrating zucchini noodles with a fresh mint, basil, and parsley pistou (*le français* for "pesto"); protein-filled gigante beans; and plenty of sweet peas for bright pops of flavor *and* tons of antiaging, immune-boosting benefits. No one would turn down a glass of chilled rosé alongside this green goddess!

1   Make the herb pistou: In a blender, combine all the ingredients and blend until smooth. Taste and add more salt, if desired. Set aside.

2   Make the pasta: In a large bowl, massage the kale in the oil with a pinch of salt until it's slightly softened and tender. Arrange the kale on a large serving plate and set aside.

3   In the same bowl, toss together the zucchini, beans, peas, and lemon juice with a pinch of salt. Gently fold in enough of the pistou to coat, then arrange the mixture on top of the plated kale and serve. This is delicious as a chilled raw noodle dish, or toss in a sauté pan for 5 to 10 minutes until warm if you prefer it heated. We like it both ways! Store the extra pistou in the fridge for up to 3 days.

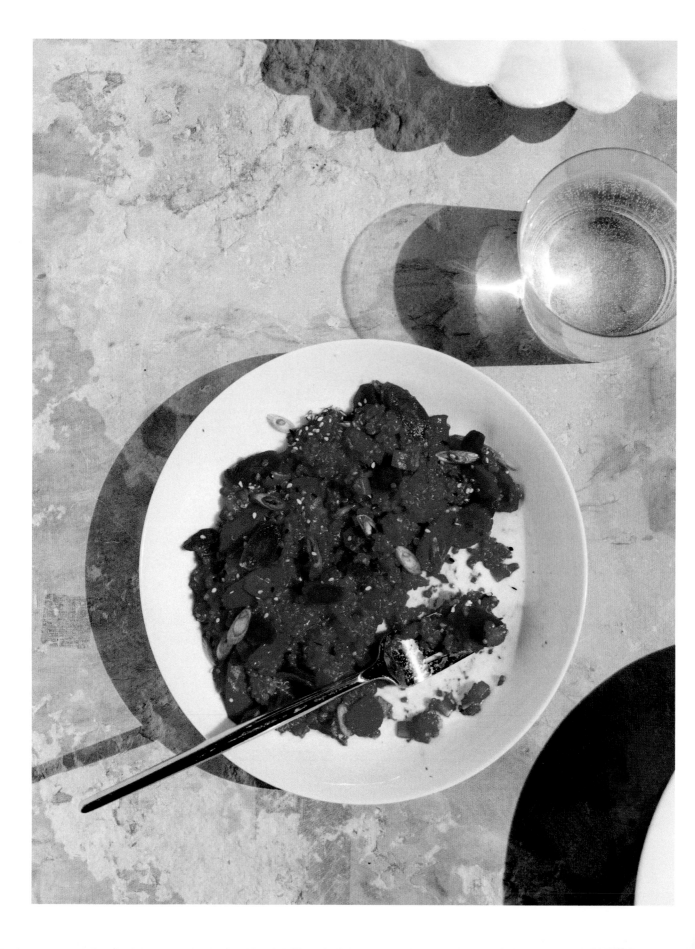

CARROT RISOTTO

SERVES 4

2 tablespoons extra-virgin
    olive oil

1 medium yellow onion,
    finely diced

4 sprigs fresh thyme, leaves
    picked

2 cloves garlic, grated or
    finely chopped

1 cup (170 g) uncooked white
    quinoa, rinsed under cold
    water for 1 minute

2 tablespoons coconut oil

2 cups (300 g) carrots, cut into
    ¼-inch (6 mm) rounds

Himalayan salt

2 tablespoons vegetable stock
    or water

2 tablespoons wildflower honey

1 tablespoon toasted sesame oil,
    plus more for serving

¼ cup (60 ml) tamari soy sauce

1 tablespoon grated fresh
    ginger

1 teaspoon ground turmeric

2 scallions (light green parts),
    thinly sliced on the bias,
    for garnish

1 tablespoon sesame seeds,
    for garnish

In our opinion, there isn't a sexier, more special occasion–suited dish than risotto. And yet, it couldn't be simpler to make at home—especially with our Sakarafied twist: subbing complete-protein quinoa for Arborio rice. Then we give the dish even more buttery body by folding in honey- and tamari-glazed carrots that have been whipped into a puree. It's fitting that carrots take center stage in this dish, as they're a particularly good source of beta-carotene, an antioxidant that the body converts into vitamin A and that is crucial for the immune system, reproductive wellness, and, above all, healthy vision—all the better for gazing into your lover's eyes. Serve with Daily Greens (page 33): perhaps sautéed kale with a bit of garlic and olive oil.

Even though we love all the colorful heirloom varieties of carrots you can now find at the market, you'll want to stick with classic orange if you want intense color in your risotto.

1   In a medium saucepot, heat the olive oil over medium-high heat. Add the onion, thyme, and garlic and sauté for 2 to 3 minutes. Add the quinoa and sauté for another 2 to 3 minutes. Add 2 cups (480 ml) of water and bring the mixture to a boil, then reduce the heat to low and cover the pot. Cook the quinoa until it has absorbed all the liquid, about 15 minutes. Remove the pot from the heat and keep it covered as you prepare the rest of the risotto.

RECIPE CONTINUES

2   In a large skillet, heat the coconut oil over medium heat. Add the carrots and sauté for 2 to 3 minutes. Season with a pinch of salt, then add the vegetable stock and 1 tablespoon of the honey. Continue cooking the carrots until the liquid thickens and the carrots are tender, about 10 minutes. Remove half of the carrots from the pot and set them aside. Add the sesame oil, tamari, ginger, turmeric, the remaining 1 tablespoon of honey and 3 tablespoons of water to the pot and bring to a simmer. Transfer the mixture to a blender or food processor and puree until completely smooth.

3   Fold the carrot puree and glazed carrots into the quinoa and garnish with the scallions and sesame seeds. Drizzle with toasted sesame oil and serve hot.

SUNSHINE CURRY STEW

Without the sun, there is no light; there is no life. This creamy and intoxicating (and detoxifying) stew gives us a burst of life that feels like it's coming directly from the sun. It's a great dish for any time of day, as, while it is filling, it won't weigh you down. It's infused with warming spices and aromatics like curry powder, turmeric, garlic, ginger, and lemongrass, which not only provide whole-body cleansing but also stir the libido, stoke the digestive fire, and give you blazing—but balanced—energy, not unlike our favorite star.

Luckily, lemongrass is becoming easier to find at your local grocery store, which means you can toss it into simmering broths, stews, and teas for a dose of its antioxidant-packing, metabolism-revving, cold- and flu-healing powers. If your store doesn't carry it, most Asian markets do.

SERVES 2

½ cup (115 g) short-grain brown rice

1 tablespoon coconut oil

½ medium yellow onion, diced

2 cloves garlic, minced

1 stalk lemongrass, outer layers peeled, core discarded, and halved

1 (1-inch/2.5 cm) knob ginger, peeled and grated

1 tablespoon yellow curry powder

2 small red chiles, such as Thai, Fresno, or jalapeño, seeded and thinly sliced (less if you don't like spice)

1 medium carrot, halved and sliced into ½-inch (12 mm) half-moons

1 large sweet potato, peeled and cut into ½-inch (12 mm) cubes

1 zucchini, halved and sliced into ½-inch (12 mm) half-moons

10 cherry tomatoes

2 cups (480 ml) coconut milk

4 cups (120 g) spinach

¼ cup (40 g) frozen peas

2 scallions (white and green parts), thinly sliced

2 sprigs fresh cilantro, roughly chopped

2 teaspoons tamari soy sauce

2 tablespoons lime juice

Himalayan salt

RECIPE CONTINUES

1　In a small saucepot, bring the rice and 1 cup (240 ml) of water to a boil. Cover the pot and reduce to low heat. Let the rice cook until it absorbs all the liquid and becomes tender, about 30 minutes. Remove from the heat and cover to keep warm. Set aside.

2　In a medium saucepot, combine the oil, onion, garlic, lemongrass, ginger, and curry powder over medium heat. Depending on how spicy you want the curry, toss in either all the sliced chiles or just a few slices. Sauté for 5 minutes, stirring frequently. Add the carrot and sweet potato and sauté for another 2 to 3 minutes. Add the zucchini and tomatoes and sauté for another 2 to 3 minutes. Stir in the milk and ½ cup (120 ml) of water and bring to a simmer. Cook for 10 to 15 minutes. Remove the lemongrass and discard. Fold in the spinach, peas, scallions, cilantro, tamari, and lime juice. Season with salt, if needed.

3　To serve, place the rice in the base of a bowl and spoon the curry mix over. Enjoy warm.

Light
WORK ▬▬▬▬▬

TAKE UP SPACE This will help you expand your light energy and take up the space you deserve in the world. *Step 1*: Speak up. At every opportunity you're given, practice speaking up. Present something at work. Say hello a little louder and prouder. Let people know you're there. *Step 2*: Stand up. Plant your feet on the ground and spread your arms wide. Imagine energy shooting like beams of light through your limbs and up through the top of your head. Stretch and feel yourself lengthen in every direction.

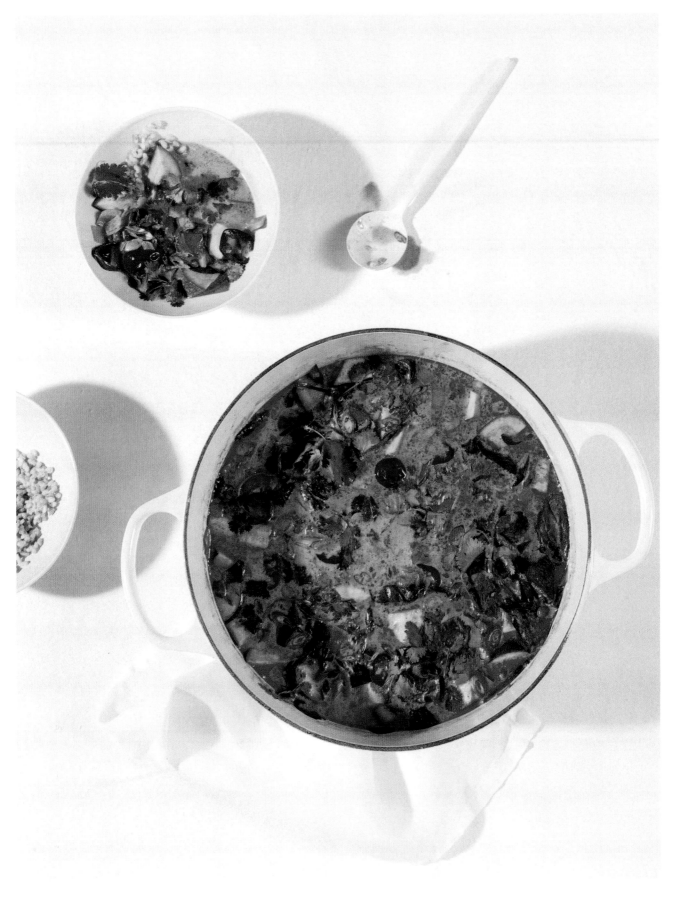

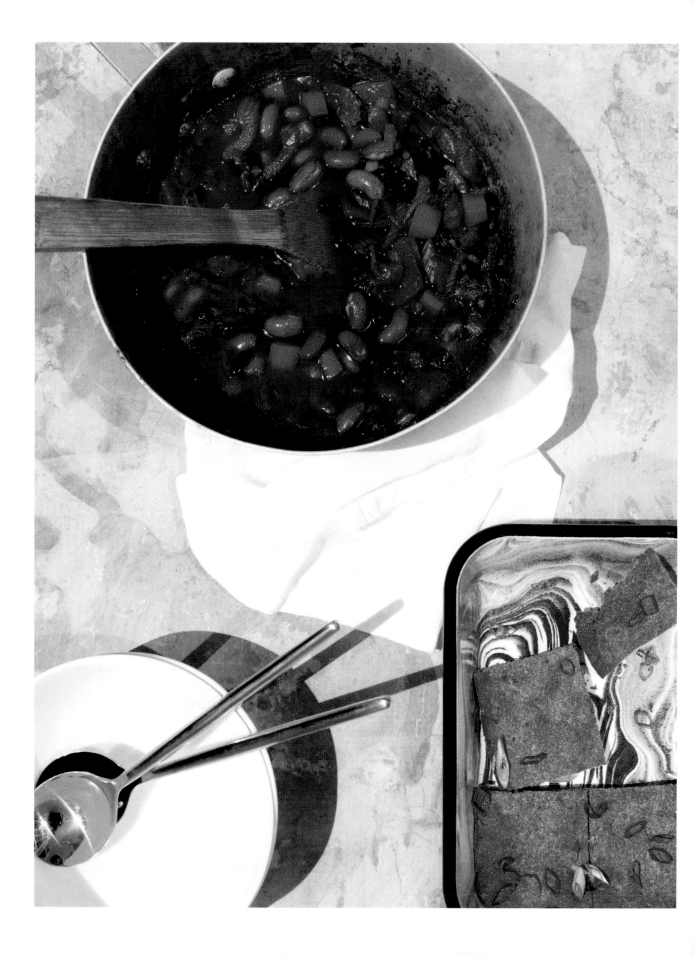

COWBOY CHILI + CORN BREAD

This chili is full of anti-inflammatory spices, muscle-building protein, and a whole lot of blood sugar–balancing (and waist-shrinking!) fiber. We use kombu in our broth, which not only imparts a deeper flavor but also infuses the chili with its vitamins and minerals. We also add in dried chiles because we like it hot, but you can substitute chipotle peppers in adobo sauce for a smokier experience. Eat it with a slice of our gluten-free (and guilt-free) corn bread and you bet your pretty pony you're going to be feeling good.

1   Make the chili: If using chiles in adobo sauce, proceed to step 2. If using dried chiles, in a small bowl, combine the chiles with just enough boiling water to cover. Soak the peppers until very soft, about 30 minutes. Remove their stems and seeds. Finely mince the chiles until they're pulpy but not quite a paste (you can also do this in a blender). Set aside.

SERVES 4

FOR THE CHILI

3 chiles in adobo sauce, rinsed and minced, or 2 dried chipotle peppers

1 small poblano pepper

1 tablespoon extra-virgin olive oil

1 cup (150 g) diced white onion (about ½ large onion)

1 cup (100 g) diced celery (about 3 stalks)

1 cup (150 g) diced carrots (about 2 medium carrots)

2 cloves garlic, minced

1 cup (170 g) cooked or canned black beans, rinsed and drained

1 cup (180 g) cooked or canned kidney beans, rinsed and drained

⅓ cup (75 ml) tomato paste

⅓ cup (20 g) packed sun-dried tomatoes, chopped

¼ cup (55 g) yellow lentils (or dal)

1 strip kombu

1 tablespoon dried oregano

2½ teaspoons tamari soy sauce

1 teaspoon fresh lemon juice

1 teaspoon ground cumin

¼ teaspoon Himalayan salt, or more to taste

FOR THE CORN BREAD

1 teaspoon coconut or extra-virgin olive oil

⅓ cup (75 ml) unsweetened applesauce

2 tablespoons unsweetened nut or hemp milk

½ cup (65 g) cornmeal

1 cup (160 g) brown rice flour

¼ cup (35 g) coconut palm sugar

1 tablespoon flaxseed meal

1½ teaspoons baking powder

½ teaspoon xanthan gum

¼ teaspoon Himalayan salt

1 tablespoon sliced scallions, for garnish

RECIPE CONTINUES

2 Preheat the broiler. Place the poblano pepper on an unlined baking sheet and broil for 2 minutes per side, or until the skin is quite blackened and blistered and the pepper has softened slightly (you can also do this over a flame on the stove top, if you have a gas range). Place the pepper in a bowl and cover with plastic wrap or a towel and let sit for 15 minutes. Once the pepper is just cool enough to handle, peel the pepper, remove the stem and seeds, and chop. Set aside.

3 In a large pot, heat the oil over medium-high heat. Add the onion, celery, carrots, and garlic and sauté for 3 minutes to sweat. Add the remaining ingredients along with the poblano pepper and chiles in adobo sauce or chipotle peppers. Stir and cook for 2 minutes before adding 4 cups (960 ml) of water. Bring the mixture to a boil, reduce to a simmer, and cook for 45 minutes, or until the vegetables and lentils are soft and the flavors have melded. Stir regularly to prevent scorching on the bottom of the pot, and if the mixture starts to get too thick, add 1 cup (240 ml) of water. Remove and discard the kombu, adding more salt, if desired, and keep warm until ready to serve.

4 Make the corn bread: Preheat the oven to 350°F (175°C). Lightly grease a 6-inch (15 cm) cast-iron skillet or small baking dish with coconut or olive oil and set side.

5 In a medium bowl, whisk together the applesauce and milk.

6 In a large bowl, combine the cornmeal, flour, sugar, flaxseed meal, baking powder, xanthan gum, and salt. Stir to combine. Stir in the wet ingredients and mix until the batter is uniform. Pour the batter into the prepared pan; it should be about ½ inch (12 mm) thick. Smooth the top with a spatula and bake for about 15 minutes, or until golden brown. Slice into 8 pieces, garnish with scallions, and serve warm.

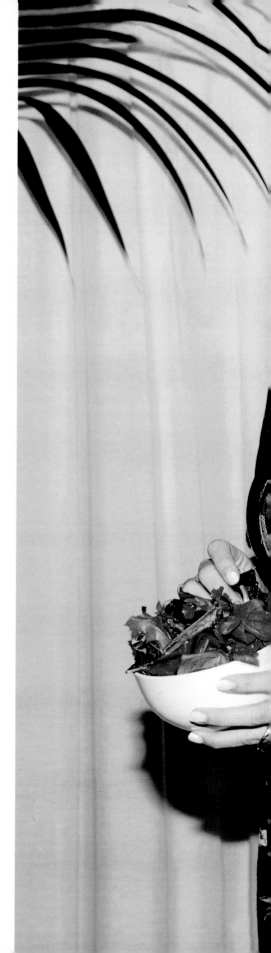

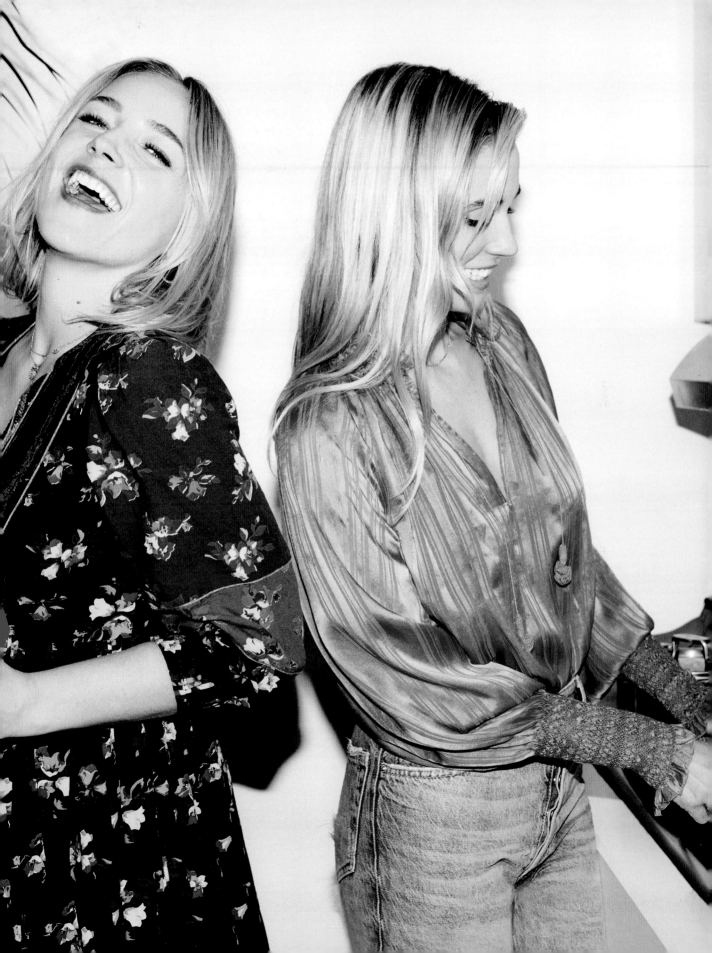

SAKARA CLASSIC CAESAR

FOR THE DRESSING

½ avocado, pitted and peeled

¼ cup (60 ml) plus 1 tablespoon fresh lemon juice

2 tablespoons nutritional yeast

1½ tablespoons hemp seeds

1 clove garlic, roughly chopped

2 teaspoons Dijon mustard

¼ teaspoon freshly ground black pepper

¼ teaspoon Himalayan salt

3½ tablespoons (52.5 ml) extra-virgin olive oil

FOR THE SALAD

1 cup (165 g) cooked or canned cannellini beans, rinsed and drained

¾ cup (85 g) Botija olives

2 teaspoons extra-virgin olive oil

1 teaspoon fresh lemon juice

12 ounces (340 g) chopped romaine lettuce

Homemade Almond "Parmesan" (page 184)

Garlic Croutons (page 116)

EAT CLEAN

It's hard to improve on perfection, but we managed to take the Caesar and make it truly fit for a conqueror. Our dressing hits all the same salty, creamy notes as the traditional version but won't weigh you down, and we finish the whole thing off with a sprinkle of our Homemade Almond "Parmesan" and a handful of garlicky, olive oil–kissed croutons made from our beloved seed bread. Romaine lettuce is one of the most hydrating foods you can eat, and, to add an extra healing element, we call for Botija olives. Many olives that you find in the store have been picked before they're fully ripe, softened with chemicals like lye, artificially darkened with an iron compound called ferrous gluconate, and pasteurized, or cooked at a high temperature to burn off any bacteria but also any remaining nutrients. We believe this sumptuous stone fruit deserves much better, and, luckily, organic Botija olives are given the royal spa treatment from the moment they're fully ripe—cured in sea salt and dried at a low temperature. The result is a tastier olive that's also rich in vitamins A and E, calcium, and oleic acid, a beneficial monounsaturated fat that supports youthful, supple skin, even on life's battlefield.

1   Make the dressing: In a blender, combine all the ingredients except the oil. Blend until smooth. With the blender running, slowly stream in the oil until the dressing is thick and emulsified.

2   To assemble: In a medium bowl, toss the beans and olives with the oil and lemon juice.

3   Arrange the lettuce in a large bowl. Top with the dressed beans and olives, parm, croutons, and dressing. Store any leftover dressing in the fridge for up to 5 days.

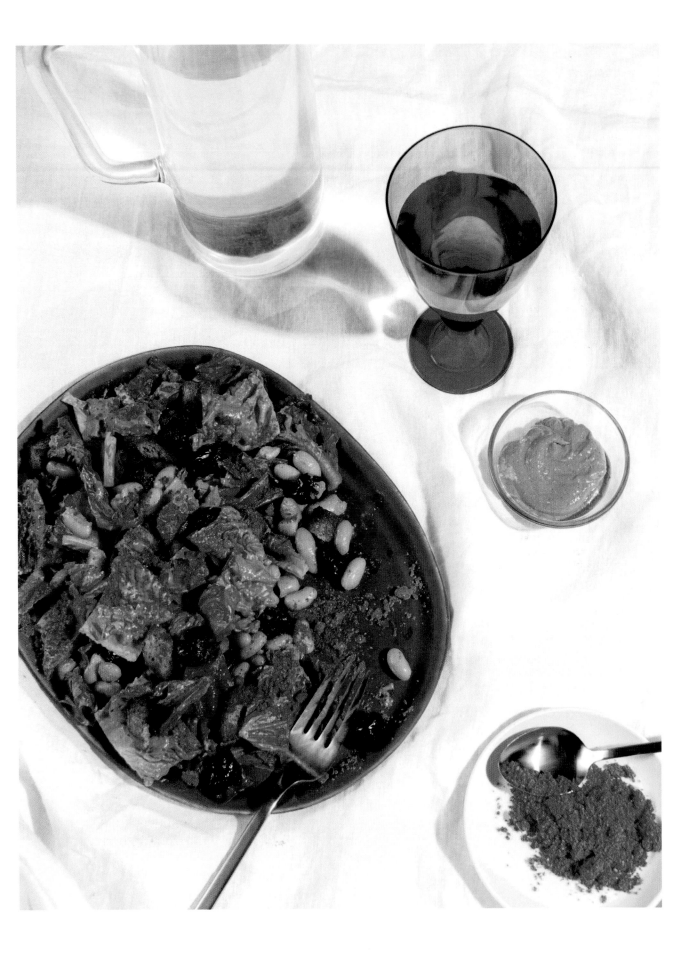

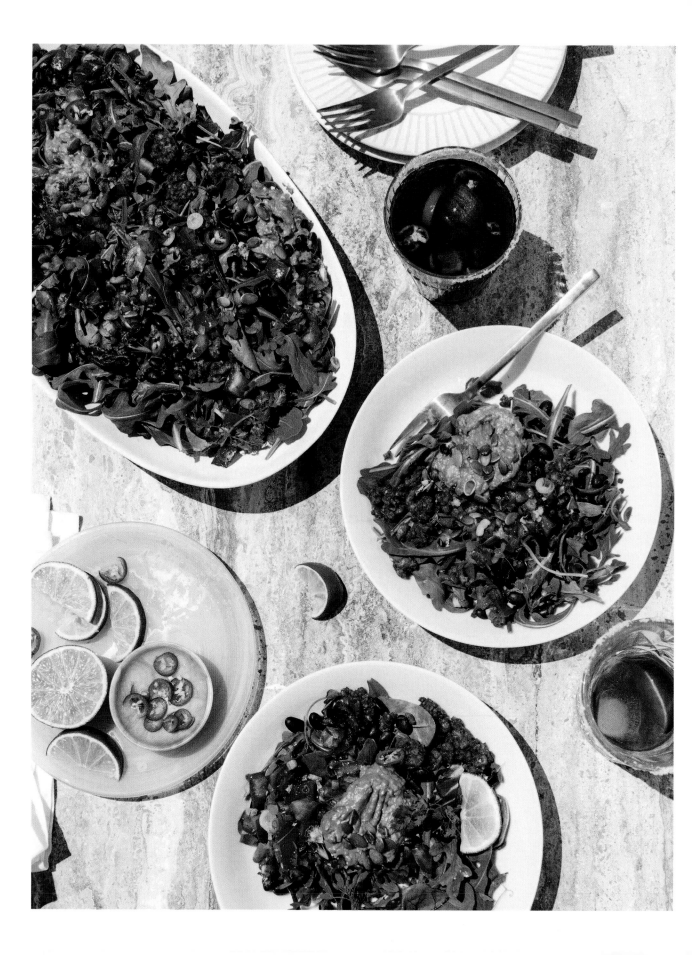

TACO SALAD WITH WALNUT "CHORIZO"

We make our taco salad with classic flavors, including homemade pico de gallo (though you could also buy a fresh version from the grocery store), but the star is a spicy walnut "chorizo" that's flavorful and satisfying. We highly recommend making a larger batch because you can store it in the fridge for up to two weeks and crumble it into wraps, sprinkle it over your Chickpea Scramble (page 44), or toss it into salads. You can serve this dish as is, or add a stack of warmed corn tortillas for instant—and *muy delicioso*—tacos.

SERVES 4

FOR THE PICO DE GALLO

4 Roma tomatoes, diced

1 large shallot, minced

2 scallions (white and light green parts), thinly sliced

2 cloves garlic, minced

¼ to ½ jalapeño (depending on how much heat you like), seeded and minced

4 sprigs fresh cilantro, leaves chopped

1 tablespoon extra-virgin olive oil

Juice of 1 lime

Himalayan salt

FOR THE WALNUT "CHORIZO"

1 cup (100 g) raw walnuts

1 teaspoon chili powder

1 teaspoon smoked paprika

½ teaspoon ground cumin

2 teaspoons tamari soy sauce

2 teaspoons fresh lime juice

1 teaspoon wildflower honey

Himalayan salt

FOR THE SALAD

2 avocados, pitted and peeled

Himalayan salt

1 cup (170 g) cooked or canned black beans, rinsed and drained

Juice of 1 lemon

12 cups (360 g) mixed greens (about two 15-ounce/455 g clamshells)

2 cups (200 g) shredded cabbage

8 sprigs fresh cilantro, leaves picked

¼ cup (35 g) pumpkin seeds

Lime wedges, for serving

RECIPE CONTINUES

1   Make the pico de gallo: In a medium bowl, combine the tomatoes, shallot, scallions, garlic, jalapeño, and cilantro and toss with the oil, lime juice, and a pinch of salt. Let the mixture marinate while you make the "chorizo" and the salad.

2   Make the "chorizo": In a food processor, combine all the ingredients with a pinch of salt and process until the mixture begins to stick to itself but isn't totally smooth. Set aside.

3   Assemble the salad: In a small bowl, mash the avocados with a pinch of salt.

4   In another small bowl, toss the black beans with the lemon juice and a pinch of salt.

5   Divide the greens and cabbage among 4 large plates. Top with the pico de gallo (juices and all), black beans (making sure to include some of the lemon juice), crumbles of the walnut "chorizo," and theavocado smash. Garnish with the cilantro leaves and pumpkin seeds and serve with lime wedges.

WALNUTS

Walnuts NOURISH THE BLOOD, *support digestion,* AND TONIFY THE KIDNEYS

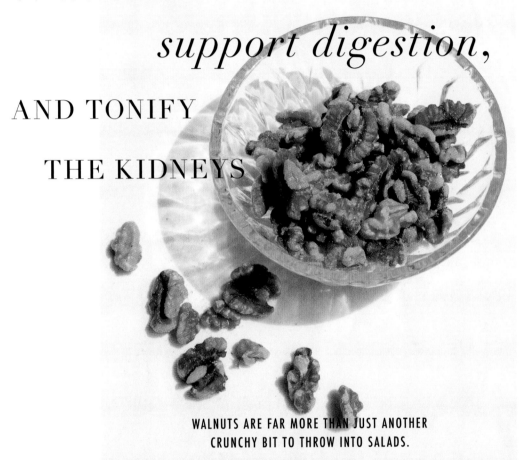

WALNUTS ARE FAR MORE THAN JUST ANOTHER CRUNCHY BIT TO THROW INTO SALADS.

As a highly regarded healing food in Chinese traditional medicine, walnuts are associated with the lung, large intestine, and kidney meridians, and are prescribed to nourish the blood, support digestion, and tonify the kidneys. (Traditional healers consider the kidneys the most important organ system because they're the keeper of chi—life energy—and are able to lend healing energy to other organs that may be depleted.) Walnuts are nutritionally potent too, containing neuroprotective compounds, or agents that protect and nourish the brain, such as vitamin E, folate, melatonin, omega-3 fatty acids, and antioxidants. In fact, eating just ¼ cup (25 grams) of walnuts provides more than 100 percent of the recommended daily amount of omega-3s, along with a big dose of copper, manganese, molybdenum, and biotin. Walnuts also contain the amino acid L-arginine, a powerful guardian of heart health.

167

CAULIFLOWER WITH COCONUT YOGURT + POMEGRANATE

1 teaspoon ground paprika

1 teaspoon ground turmeric powder

1 teaspoon ground cumin

1 teaspoon ground coriander

1 teaspoon Himalayan salt, or more to taste

½ teaspoon coconut palm sugar

½ teaspoon cayenne pepper

¼ cup (60 ml) coconut oil, melted

1 head cauliflower, stem trimmed, leaves left attached

2 small red onions, thinly sliced

½ cup (120 ml) Orgasmic Coconut Yogurt (page 62) or store-bought

Juice of ½ lemon

½ small cucumber, sliced thin

1 cup (175 g) pomegranate seeds

Cruciferous veggies like kale, cauliflower, and cabbage provide sulfur, a building block of every metabolic reaction in your body that's also a cleansing, energizing agent, helping the liver and kidneys to fend off toxins and fuel the mitochondria (or energy centers) in your cells. And sulfur is required for the creation of keratin, which is needed for lustrous, supple hair and skin, and strong nails. But what we're most excited about is how tender, caramelized, and downright meaty a whole head of cauli gets when you slather it with warming spices like turmeric, paprika, cumin, and coriander and roast it as-is (no messy chopping required). Sprinkle it with pomegranate arils and add a drizzle of coconut yogurt sauce and you have a special occasion centerpiece.

1   Preheat the oven to 350°F (175°C). Line a baking sheet with parchment paper and set aside.

2   In a medium bowl, stir together the paprika, turmeric, cumin, coriander, salt, sugar, and cayenne. Whisk in the oil, creating a paste. Set aside 1 teaspoon of the mixture.

3   Place the cauliflower on one half of the baking sheet and spread the onions over the other half. Slather everything with the spice mixture, making sure to get into all the nooks and crannies of the cauliflower. Roast until the onions are tender and caramelized, 25 to 30 minutes. Remove the onions and continue roasting the cauliflower for another 20 to 30 minutes.

4   Allow the cauliflower to cool slightly before slicing into wedges.

5   In a small bowl, stir together the yogurt, reserved spice paste, and lemon juice. Top with the cucumber slices. Top the cauliflower with the caramelized onion and pomegranate seeds and serve with the spiced coconut yogurt.

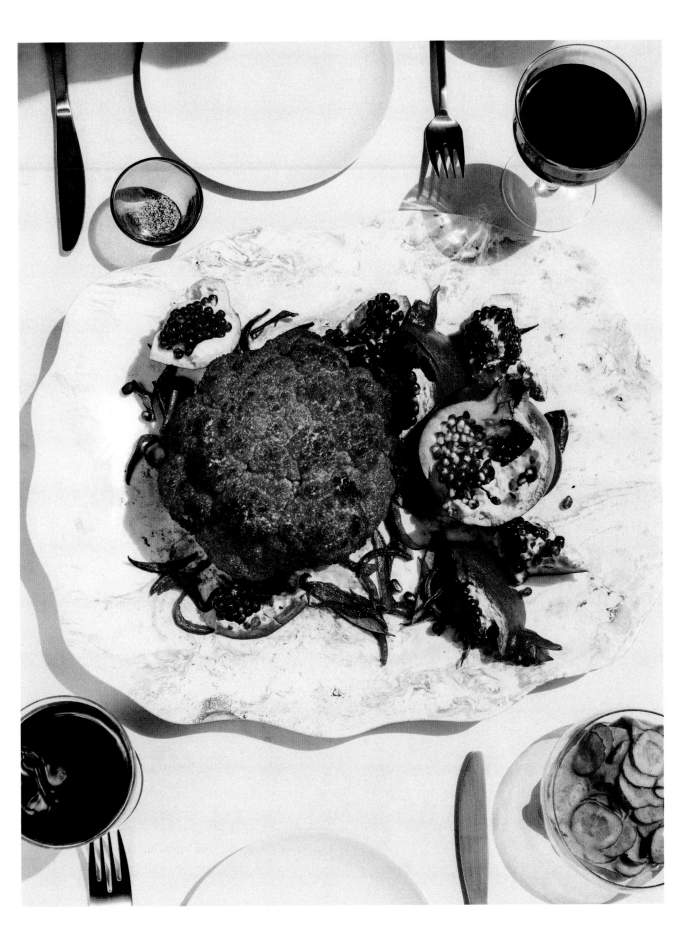

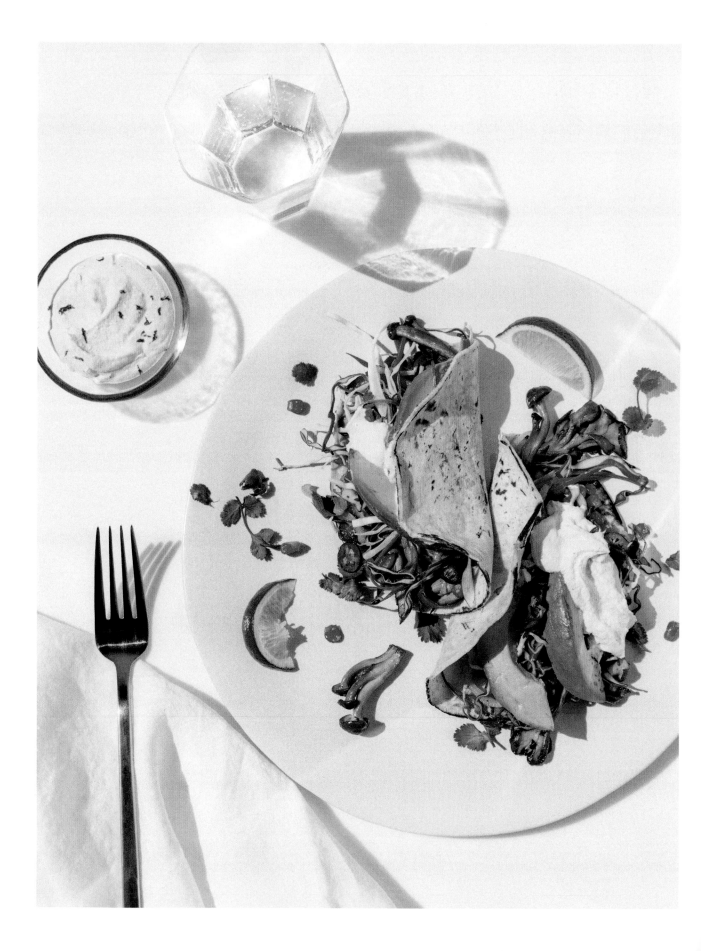

WILD MUSHROOM + CORN TACOS WITH SPICY SLAW AND CASHEW CREMA

SERVES 4

You can take the girl out of Arizona, but you can't take Arizona out of the girl! Tacos are a pretty essential part of our diets, which is why one of our first Sakara missions was coming up with a version that would satisfy our love for a taco without weighing us down. We love how versatile this recipe is—like the LBD of dishes.

FOR THE CASHEW CREMA

1 cup (120 g) raw cashews, soaked overnight and drained

Juice of 1 lime

½ teaspoon cayenne pepper (less if you don't like spice)

¼ teaspoon Himalayan salt

FOR THE SPICY SLAW

¼ small head purple cabbage, shredded

¼ small head green cabbage, shredded

1 medium carrot, shredded

½ cup (25 g) fresh cilantro leaves, roughly chopped

½ jalapeño, seeded and thinly sliced

Juice of ½ lime

1 teaspoon Himalayan salt

FOR THE WILD MUSHROOM AND CORN FILLING

2 tablespoons extra-virgin olive oil

1 shallot, sliced

4 cloves garlic, sliced

8 ounces (about 4 cups/500 g) wild mushrooms, such as shiitake, maitake, or oyster, wiped clean with a damp cloth and cut into bite-size pieces

Himalayan salt

1 cup (175 g) sweet corn kernels, fresh or frozen

FOR SERVING

8 corn tortillas

2 avocados, pitted and sliced

Fresh cilantro, for garnish

RECIPE CONTINUES

1   Make the cashew crema: In a blender or food processor, combine the cashews, lime juice, cayenne, and salt with ¼ cup (60 ml) of water. Blend until smooth. Taste and add more salt, if desired. Transfer the crema to a serving bowl and set aside.

2   Make the spicy slaw: In a medium bowl, toss together the cabbage, carrot, cilantro, jalapeño, lime juice, and salt. Set aside.

3   Make the wild mushroom and corn filling: In a large pan, heat the olive oil over medium heat. Add the shallot and garlic and cook until the shallot is translucent and the garlic hasn't yet begun to brown, 1 to 2 minutes. Add the mushrooms, season with a pinch of salt, and cook until tender, 7 to 8 minutes. Add the corn and cook for another 2 minutes. Taste the filling and add more salt, if desired.

4   Serve: Using a pair of tongs and working in batches, char the tortillas over an open flame on the stove until they are just taking on color and warmed through. Keep the finished tortillas under a clean towel so they'll stay warm. Serve the tortillas with the filling, slaw, and crema, plus slices of avocado and fresh cilantro.

MUSHROOMS

Tap into THE WISEST PLANT SPECIES *on the planet*

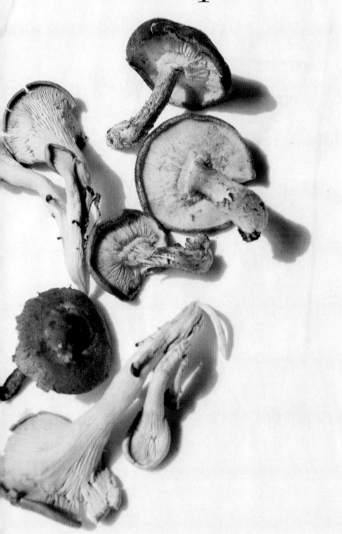

MUSHROOMS ARE ONE OF THE MOST NUTRIENT-DENSE, VITAMIN-RICH, LIFE-GIVING, ULTRAHEALING MEDICINAL FOODS YOU CAN FIND AT THE MARKET.

Think about it: Fungi are pretty invincible, spanning millions of years and surviving a vast variety of ecosystems and climate changes, surpassing the dinosaurs and able to exist underwater and in outer space. When we consume foods with that caliber of evolutionary prowess, we are ingesting something incredibly beneficial to our bodies, which is why most, if not all, ancient civilizations have admired the mushroom. We also now know that mushrooms are among the wisest plant species on our planet. Thanks to the mycelium, or the mass of thin threads that makes up their bodies, mushrooms can create an underground communication network that isn't unlike the Internet. The roots of plants and trees can tap into this network, allowing them to create community, share nutrients and resources, and eliminate potentially harmful soil invaders. When we eat mushrooms, we're providing our bodies with major health benefits: They're one of the only edible sources of vitamin D (crucial for neurological, endocrine, and lymphatic health), and they can lower blood pressure, provide ample fiber and folate (essential for preventing iron deficiency), and even combat certain cancers. But we'd also like to think that by eating these miraculous plants we're also tapping into the neural network and age-old wisdom of the earth.

DINNER

173

ROASTED ARTICHOKE + CARAMELIZED ONION GALETTE

**FOR THE ARTICHOKE
AND ONION FILLING**

2 medium yellow onions,
 quartered

4 cloves garlic

1 cup (170 g) canned organic
 artichoke hearts, drained

4 sprigs fresh thyme

½ cup (120 ml) extra-virgin
 olive oil

Himalayan salt and freshly
 ground black pepper

1 pound (.5 kg) baby spinach
 leaves

FOR THE CRUST

1 tablespoon extra-virgin
 olive oil

1 cup (158 g) brown rice flour

½ cup (45 g) chickpea flour

½ cup (60 g) buckwheat flour
 or all-purpose gluten-free
 flour

¼ cup (30 g) arrowroot powder

Pinch of Himalayan salt

2 tablespoons coconut palm
 sugar

¼ cup (60 ml) coconut oil,
 melted

¼ cup (60 ml) extra-virgin
 olive oil or melted ghee,
 plus extra for the pan

¼ cup (60 ml) apple cider
 vinegar

There's something so effortlessly cool about a perfectly imperfect galette—essentially, a free-form pie—whether it's served up simply for lunch with a side of greens or as part of a polished dinner spread. The gluten-free crust we use here features some of our favorite earthy, nutty flours (chickpea, brown rice, buckwheat) and is an all-around staple. You can use it as the base for any savory tart, pie, or even pizza, layering it with whatever pureed, roasted, or grilled goodness you're in the mood for. This recipe makes enough for two crusts, so stash the leftovers in the fridge for up to two days, or in the freezer for up to two weeks. Just thaw it or bring it to room temperature before rolling it out and celebrating the rustic, the rumpled, and all things charming in their imperfection.

1 Make the filling: Preheat the oven to 400°F (205°C).

2 Arrange the onions, garlic, artichoke hearts, and thyme on a large baking sheet. Drizzle with the olive oil and sprinkle with salt and pepper. Toss to evenly coat. Bake for 15 minutes, remove the garlic and set aside, then bake for another 15 minutes, or until the onions and artichokes are tender and golden.

3 Place half of the mixture, including the garlic, in a food processor and pulse until slightly chunky. In a large bowl, stir together the puree with the other half of the mixture. Fold in the spinach and allow to cool while you make the crust.

4 Make the crust: Preheat the oven to 350°F (175°C). Lightly grease a 10-inch (25 cm) pie pan with olive oil and set aside.

RECIPE CONTINUES

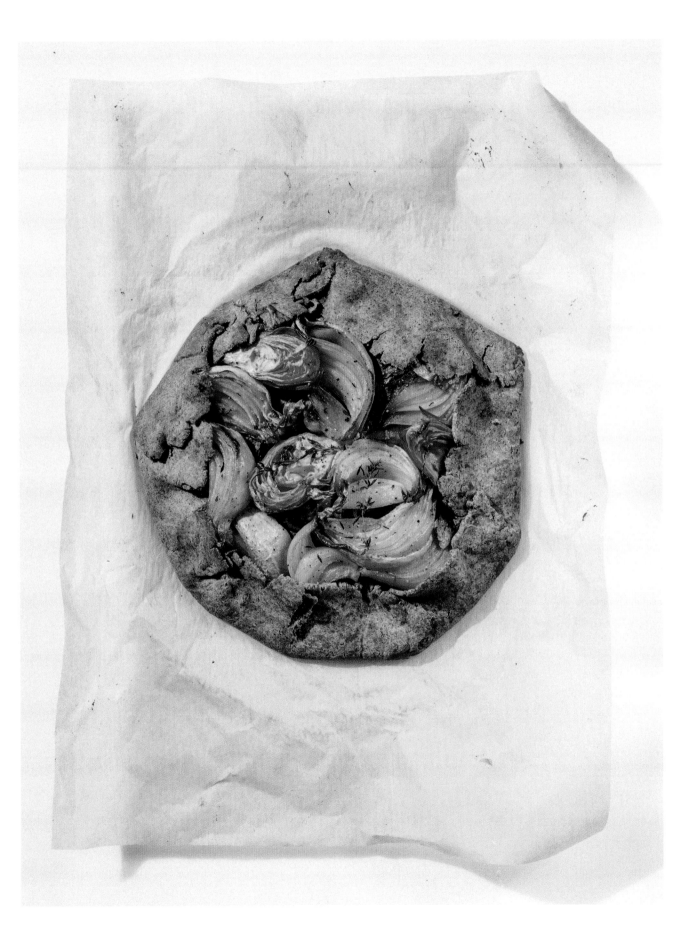

5   In the bowl of a stand mixer fitted with the paddle attachment, combine the flours, arrowroot powder, salt, and sugar.

6   In a medium bowl, combine the coconut oil, olive oil or ghee, vinegar, and ½ cup (120 ml) of water. Slowly pour the oil mixture into the dry ingredients and mix until the dough comes together. It will be a little moist. Divide the dough in half and wrap half of the dough in plastic to store in the fridge or freezer for future use.

7   Layer the remaining half of the dough between two sheets of parchment paper. Roll out the dough to about ¼ inch (6 mm) thick. It's okay if the crust isn't perfectly round! Carefully transfer the dough to the prepared pie pan and bake for 20 minutes, or until golden brown.

8   Allow the crust to cool slightly before spreading it with the filling. Leave a 1-inch (2.5 cm) border of crust around the edges. Fold the edges over the filling (it's okay if they overlap) and bake the pie for another 30 minutes, or until the filling is bubbly and golden. Serve warm or at room temperature.

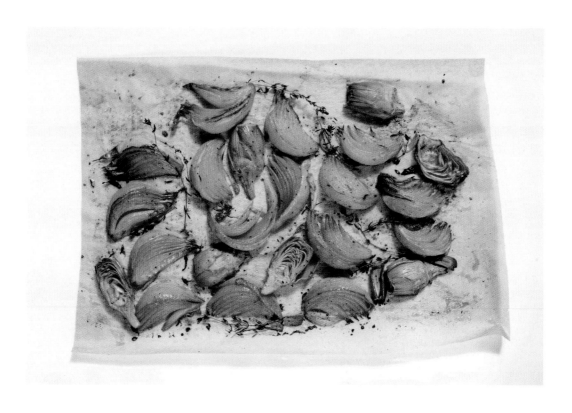

CHICKPEA WRAPS WITH SPICED WALNUT SPREAD + GRILLED AVOCADO SALSA

We love breaking out this impressive (but crazy simple) recipe for company because it takes no time to whip up a batch of warm, doughy chickpea wraps, and everyone can scoop and fill them to their heart's content. As for toppings, pretty much anything goes, but we're partial to a chili-spiced walnut spread layered with a surprising twist on an avocado salsa—grilled! Avocado, especially when it hasn't gone too ripe, chars really nicely, giving the whole dish a sultry, smoky flavor that's perfect for a summer barbecue.

SERVES 4

FOR THE SPICED WALNUT SPREAD

1 cup (100 g) raw walnuts, soaked overnight and drained

1 tablespoon nutritional yeast

1 teaspoon chili powder

1 teaspoon garlic powder

1 teaspoon onion powder

1 teaspoon smoked salt, or more to taste

Juice of ½ lime

FOR THE GRILLED AVOCADO SALSA

2 large just-ripe avocados, pitted and halved

3 tablespoons extra-virgin olive oil

1 cup (150 g) cherry tomatoes, halved

½ cup (25 g) chopped cilantro

Juice of ½ lime, or more to taste

½ teaspoon Himalayan salt, or more to taste

FOR THE CHICKPEA WRAPS

½ cup (45 g) chickpea flour

¼ teaspoon baking powder

¼ teaspoon garlic powder

¼ teaspoon Himalayan salt

⅛ teaspoon freshly ground black pepper

Extra-virgin olive oil or coconut oil

Pickled red onions (page 47)

Cilantro, for garnish

RECIPE CONTINUES

1   Make the spiced walnut spread: In a blender or food processor, combine all the ingredients and pulse until you have a chunky mixture. Taste and add more salt, if desired. Set aside.

2   Make the grilled avocado salsa: Preheat the grill or a grill pan to medium-high heat. Lightly coat the avocados with about 1 tablespoon of the oil. Place the avocados meat side down on the grill pan and cook until grill marks form, 2 to 5 minutes. Remove from the heat. Carefully peel the avocados and slice the meat into cubes.

3   In a large bowl, gently toss the grilled avocado with the tomatoes, cilantro, the remaining 2 tablespoons of oil, lime juice, and salt. Taste and adjust the seasoning with salt and/or lime juice, if desired. Set aside.

4   Make the wraps: In a small bowl, whisk together the flour, baking powder, garlic powder, salt, and pepper. Add 1 cup (240 ml) plus 2 tablespoons of water and whisk well until no clumps remain.

5   In a large pan, heat 2 tablespoons of oil over medium heat. Dropping 2 tablespoons of batter at a time, create 2 to 3 small pancakes in the pan. Cook for 1 to 2 minutes, or until bubbles form in the batter and the edges have begun to brown. Flip and cook for 1 to 2 minutes more, or until golden brown. Transfer the finished wraps to a paper towel–lined plate. Repeat with the remaining batter, adding more oil to the pan between each batch. Serve warm with the walnut spread, avocado salsa, pickled red onions, and cilantro.

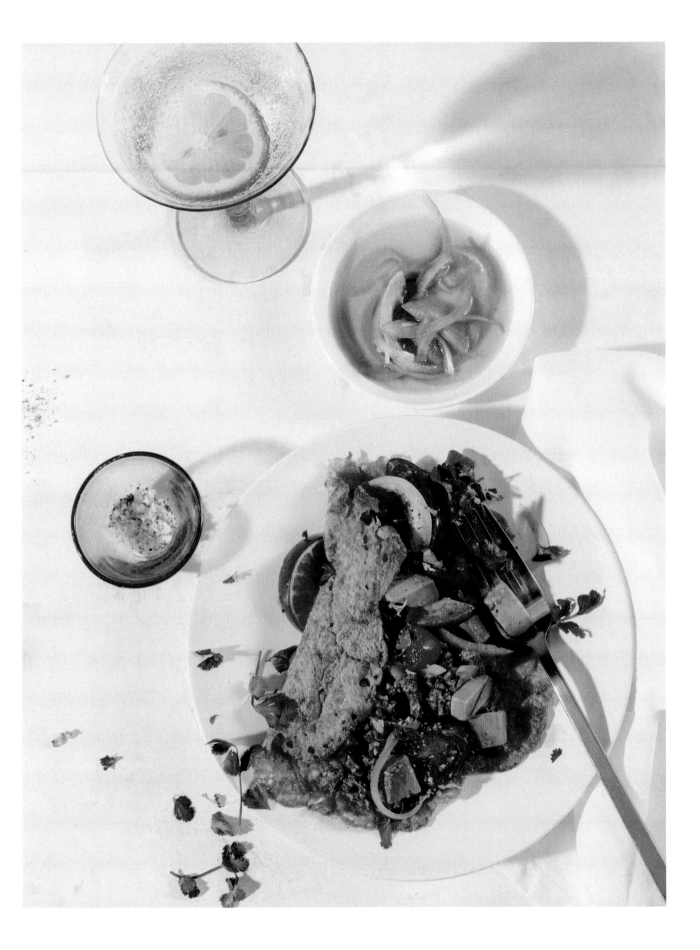

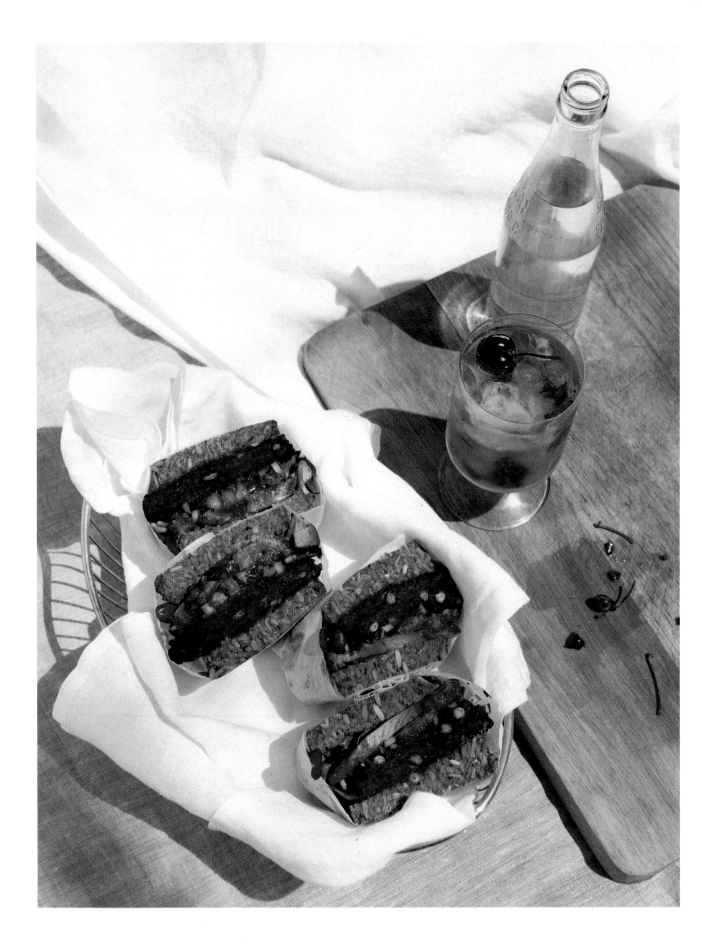

RED BEET BURGERS

Our clients are constantly asking us for our recipes (you asked; we listened!), and this is one of the most frequently requested. This burger is designed to, like a beet, root you to the earth. The betalain pigments in beets support your liver in eliminating toxins. The enzyme family glutathione S-transferases (GSTs) hooks up harmful toxins with glutathione for neutralization and elimination. We mixed these beautiful root veggies with black beans, sunflower seeds, and almonds for an extra boost of plant protein and to satisfy even your deepest hungers. Great for days when you need to detox from the craziness of daily life and get re-grounded to the earth. Eat and repeat: *Calm. Cool. Collected. I feel peace.*

SERVES 8

FOR THE BURGERS

2½ tablespoons flaxseed meal

1 cup (150 g) grated carrots (about 2 medium carrots)

1 cup (150 g) shredded beets (about ½ medium beet)

1 cup (170 g) cooked black beans, rinsed and roughly pureed or mashed

1 cup (90 g) ground oats or oat flour

½ cup (75 g) chopped yellow onion (about ½ small onion)

½ cup (70 g) sunflower seeds

⅓ cup (45 g) almonds, chopped

¼ cup (10 g) packed chopped fresh parsley

1 large clove garlic, chopped

1 tablespoon extra-virgin olive oil

1 tablespoon tamari soy sauce

1½ teaspoons chili powder

1 teaspoon ground cumin

1 teaspoon dried oregano

½ teaspoon Himalayan salt

½ teaspoon freshly ground black pepper

FOR FINISHING

1 batch Sakara Seed Bread (page 187) or your favorite store-bought buns

2 large tomatoes, sliced

1 large red onion, sliced

2 avocados, pitted and sliced

2 cups (65 g) sunflower sprouts

RECIPE CONTINUES

1   Make the burgers: Preheat the oven to 350°F (175°C). Line a baking sheet with parchment paper and set aside.

2   In a small bowl, mix the flaxseed with ½ cup (120 ml) of warm water. Let the mixture sit for 10 minutes to thicken.

3   In a food processor, combine the carrots, beets, beans, oats or oat flour, onion, sunflower seeds, almonds, parsley, garlic, oil, tamari, chili powder, cumin, oregano, salt, pepper, and flaxseed mixture. Process until the mixture is uniform and let it rest for 5 to 6 minutes at room temperature. Form the mixture into 8 tightly packed patties and arrange them on the prepared baking sheet. Bake for 20 minutes, or until the burgers are crisp on the outside and hot in the center.

4   Assemble the burgers: Top 8 slices of the bread with a patty, a slice of tomato, a slice of onion, a slice of avocado, and a handful of sprouts. Top each with another slice of bread. Serve with Daily Greens (page 33) and a drizzle of Poppy Seed Dressing (page 203).

BEETS

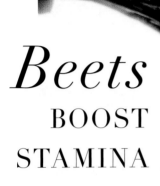

Beets

BOOST
STAMINA

FOR *every*
TYPE OF
WORKOUT

DINNER

**THE BEETROOT GROWS DEEP BENEATH THE GROUND,
SURROUNDED BY THE SOIL'S ABUNDANCE OF NUTRIENTS.**

When we eat beets, we get to tap into their grounding energy, as well as their rich stores of bioavailable benefits. The red and yellow betalain pigments in beets support the body's natural detoxification processes, helping to cleanse the blood and nourish the liver. Beets are also rich in glutathione S-transferases (GSTs), enzymes that are programmed to seek out damaging toxins, then neutralize and eliminate them. These sturdy roots contain a healthy dose of essential folate, fiber, iron, vitamin C, potassium, and manganese; and they boost stamina (beet juice is a great preworkout power-up), fight inflammation, and strengthen bones.

183

WILD MUSHROOM PASTA

SERVES 4

FOR THE HOMEMADE ALMOND "PARMESAN"

1 tablespoon raw almonds

1 tablespoon sunflower seeds

1 teaspoon nutritional yeast

¼ teaspoon smoked paprika

¼ teaspoon ground turmeric powder

¼ teaspoon Himalayan salt

FOR THE PASTA

2 cups (250 g) shiitake mushrooms, stems removed and caps roughly chopped

1 large maitake mushroom, large stem trimmed and pulled apart into bite-size pieces

1 cluster beech mushrooms, stem trimmed

2 tablespoons black truffle oil

½ teaspoon Himalayan salt, or more to taste

1 tablespoon extra-virgin olive oil

8 cups (240 g) baby spinach

1 (8-ounce/230 g) box chickpea penne

1 cup (50 g) chopped fresh parsley

1 cup (20 g) fresh basil leaves, sliced into ribbons

2 tablespoons fresh lemon juice

2 cloves garlic, minced

You might call this pasta dish a Sakara family recipe because it was created by our chef Tyler on our team's annual retreat and was loved so much by everyone that it made its way onto the menu. Its medley of wild mushrooms, fresh herbs, homemade almond–sunflower seed parmesan cheese, and deep, earthy truffle oil always brings us back to those magical moments when we pause our work and come together to talk, listen, and, of course, eat. We believe in the power of food to awaken the mind, warm the heart, and tap into our cherished shared histories. As civil rights activist Cesar Chavez said, "The people who give you their food give you their heart." We hope you can feel every ounce of our love in this dish, from our family to yours.

1   Make the parmesan: Combine all the ingredients in a blender and blend until they form a fine powder. Set aside.

2   Make the pasta: Preheat the oven to 400°F (205°C).

3   In a medium bowl, toss the mushrooms with the truffle oil and salt. Arrange the mushrooms on a baking sheet and roast for about 15 minutes, or until the mushrooms are golden brown and just beginning to crisp. Set aside.

4   In a large skillet, heat the olive oil over medium-high heat. Sauté the spinach until just wilted, about 3 minutes, and season it with a pinch of salt. Transfer the spinach to a colander to drain any excess liquid.

5   Bring a medium pot of water to a boil with a pinch of salt. Cook the pasta according to the package instructions. Drain the pasta and transfer it to a large bowl. Add the mushrooms, spinach, and parmesan and toss to combine. Top with the parsley, basil, lemon juice, and garlic and toss again, adding salt to taste, if desired. Eat with all the love in your heart.

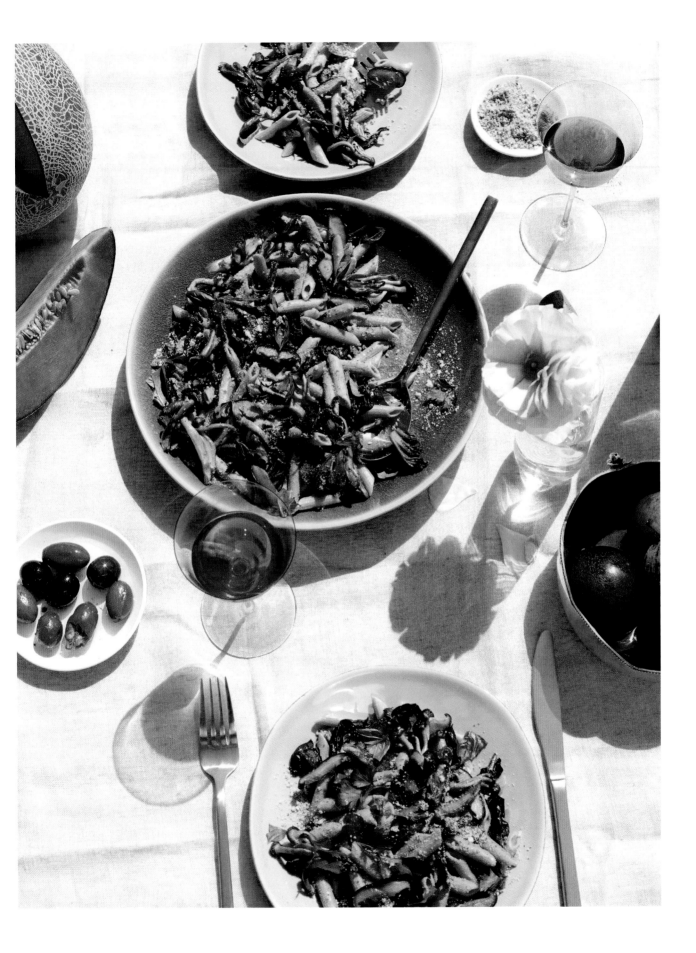

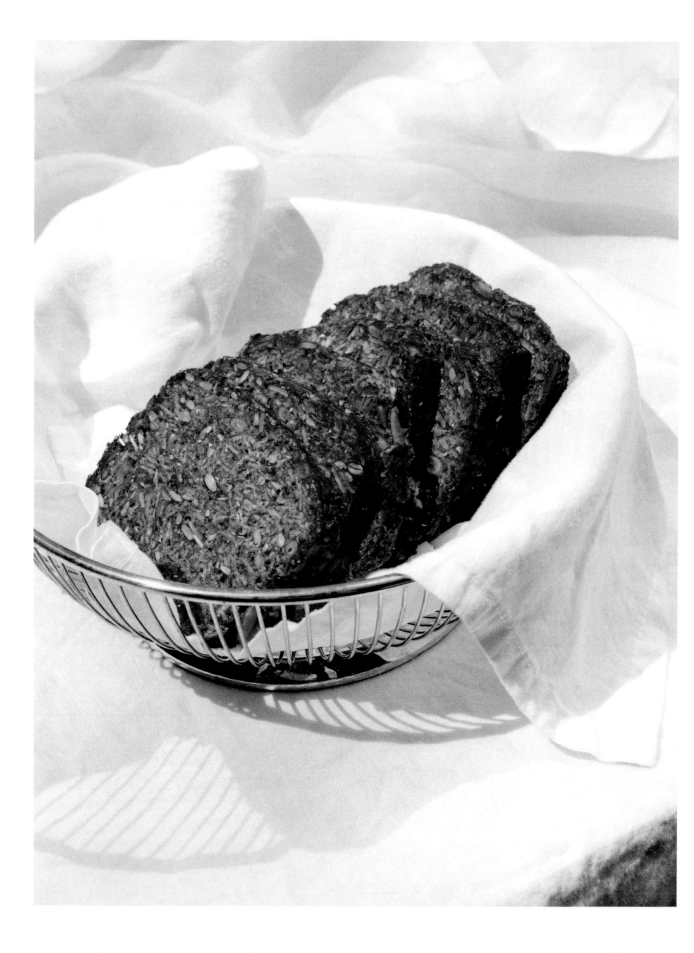

SAKARA SEED BREAD

MAKES 3 LOAVES

6 cups (540 g) gluten-free
  rolled oats

2 cups (280 g) sunflower seeds

1½ cups (145 g) sliced almonds

1¼ cups (165 g) flaxseed meal

1 cup (80 g) psyllium husk
  powder

½ cup (65 g) pumpkin seeds

½ cup (65 g) pine nuts

½ cup (80 g) chia seeds

½ cup (75 g) white sesame
  seeds

1 tablespoon Himalayan salt

½ cup (120 ml) plus
  2 tablespoons extra-virgin
  olive oil, plus 1 tablespoon
  for greasing the pan

2½ tablespoons wildflower
  honey

There are few things that are as satisfying to the soul as baking your own bread. Luckily, this oat-based, seed- and nut-packed version doesn't require hours of proofing and kneading. Our dense, chewy bread is perfect for just about any of your toast needs, whether it's the foundation of a simple breakfast or lunch, crisped up for croutons, or laid alongside a beautiful appetizer spread. This recipe makes three loaves, which is ideal because the bread freezes really nicely. Store it sliced, and all you need to do is pop it in the oven or toaster to bring it back to life.

1   In a large bowl, stir together the oats, sunflower seeds, almonds, flaxseed meal, psyllium husk powder, pumpkin seeds, pine nuts, chia seeds, sesame seeds, and salt. Fold in the oil and honey to coat, then slowly stir in 4 cups (960 ml) of water. Stir until the entire mixture is moistened. Cover the bowl with plastic wrap and let the dough rest for 30 minutes.

2   Preheat the oven to 350°F (175°C). Lightly grease an 8 by 4½-inch (20 by 11 cm) loaf pan with the oil and set aside. (You'll have enough dough for 3 loaves, so if you have more than 1 loaf pan, grease them too!)

3   Leaving about 1 inch (2.5 cm) at the top of the pan, tightly pack the dough into the prepared pan, using your hands to press it down firmly. Bake for 45 minutes, or until the crust is golden brown. Let the bread cool in the pan for 5 minutes, then turn out the loaf on a cooling rack to cool completely. Cut into ¼-inch-thick (6 mm) slices and enjoy. Store leftover bread wrapped in plastic in the fridge for up to 5 days, or in the freezer for up to 1 month.

187

THAI BURGER + ROOT FRIES

We've taken some of our favorite bold Thai flavors—garlic, ginger, cilantro, lime—and paired them with vibrant purple yams to create a bright, fresh take on a burger. Serve up these intensely satisfying sliders loaded with a larb-style cabbage and cilantro slaw and crispy sweet potato and taro root fries. Known as "the potato of the tropics," taro is native to Southeast Asia, among other places, and is rich in nutrients like magnesium, iron, manganese, zinc, and copper, as well as vitamins A, B_6, C, and E. But this grounding tuber is also extremely rich in fiber, which is essential for your digestive health.

SERVES 4

FOR THE ROOT FRIES

1 medium sweet potato, quartered lengthwise and sliced into ¾-inch-thick (2 cm) spears

1 medium taro root, halved and cut into ¾-inch-thick (2 cm) slices

1 tablespoon extra-virgin olive oil

2 tablespoons cornmeal

1¼ teaspoons Himalayan salt

FOR THE PATTIES

2 tablespoons flaxseed meal

2 teaspoons extra-virgin olive oil

1 cup (100 g) shredded purple cabbage

¼ cup (165 g) cooked or canned chickpeas, drained and rinsed

1 small purple sweet potato, peeled and grated

¼ cup (65 g) plus 2 tablespoons cooked sweet white rice or forbidden rice

2 tablespoons agar-agar

1 sprig fresh basil, roughly chopped

1 tablespoon roughly chopped fresh cilantro leaves

1 tablespoon minced fresh ginger

1 clove garlic, minced

2 teaspoons tahini

1½ teaspoons Himalayan salt, or more to taste

1¼ teaspoons extra-virgin olive oil

1 teaspoon fresh lime juice

1 teaspoon toasted sesame oil

1 teaspoon ground cumin

FOR FINISHING

3 cups (300 g) shredded purple cabbage

1 small bunch fresh cilantro, leaves roughly chopped

Tamari + Lime Vinaigrette (page 201)

Sakara Seed Bread (page 187), or your favorite gluten-free bun

RECIPE CONTINUES

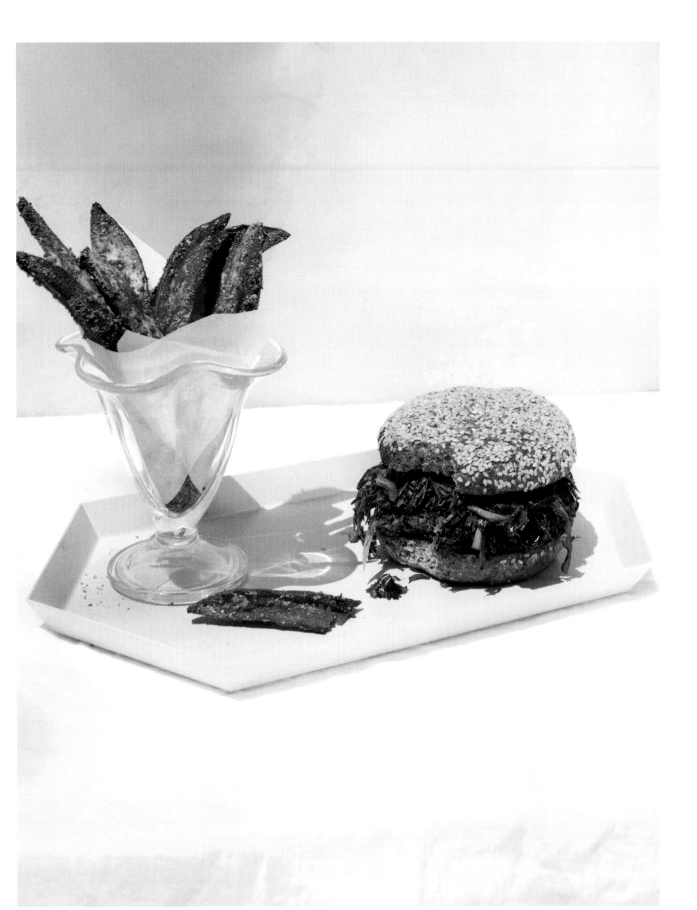

1   Make the fries: Preheat the oven to 400°F (205°C). In a large bowl, toss the sweet potatoes and taro with the oil, cornmeal, and salt. Arrange the fries in a single layer on a baking sheet. Roast for 30 to 35 minutes, flipping halfway through, until tender and lightly browned.

2   Make the patties: Mix the flaxseed meal with 3 tablespoons of water and set aside to thicken, about 10 minutes.

3   In a large skillet, heat the oil over medium heat and sauté the cabbage until tender, about 2 minutes. Set aside.

4   In a food processor or blender, pulse the chickpeas until they have the consistency of a crumbly meal.

5   Preheat the oven to 350°F (175°C). In a large bowl, combine the sautéed cabbage and the crumbled chickpeas with the flaxseed meal mixture and all the remaining ingredients. Stir to combine. Taste the mixture and add more salt, if necessary. Form the mixture into four 1-inch-thick (2.5 cm) patties and arrange them on a baking sheet. Bake for 40 minutes, or until heated through and crisp on the outside.

6   Assemble the burgers: In a large bowl, toss the cabbage and cilantro with enough dressing to coat. Let the slaw marinate for 15 minutes before serving.

7   Top 4 slices of the bread with a patty and some slaw. Finish with the remaining 4 slices of bread and serve with the fries.

MOROCCAN NIGHTS TAGINE

Tagine, a traditional Moroccan dish, is named after the special earthenware vessel that gently steams a fragrant stew of vegetables, spices, and dried fruit while melding the layers of flavors. Luckily, you don't need a tagine to feel like you're walking through the streets of Casablanca. With its cumin- and coriander-crusted sweet potatoes, cauliflower, and eggplant simmered in a bath of spiced tomatoes, chickpeas, and dried apricot gems, this heady dish is as transporting as it is healing.

SERVES 4

FOR THE QUINOA AND SPICED VEGETABLES

2 teaspoons ground cumin

1 teaspoon ground coriander

1 teaspoon ground ginger

¼ teaspoon cayenne pepper

½ teaspoon freshly ground black pepper

1 head cauliflower, broken into bite-size florets

1 medium eggplant, diced into 1-inch (2.5 cm) cubes

1 medium sweet potato, diced into 1-inch (2.5 cm) cubes

3 tablespoons extra-virgin olive oil

1 cup (170 g) uncooked quinoa

FOR THE SAUCE

1 tablespoon extra-virgin olive oil

1 medium yellow onion, diced

1 large carrot, halved and cut into ¼-inch (6 mm) half-moons

3 cloves garlic, minced

1 teaspoon Himalayan salt, or more to taste

1 (12-ounce/340 g) can chopped plum tomatoes

¼ cup (15 g) fresh cilantro leaves, roughly chopped, plus more for garnish

¼ cup (15 g) fresh parsley leaves, roughly chopped

1 teaspoon ground turmeric

8 cups (240 g) baby kale

1 cup (165 g) cooked or canned chickpeas, rinsed and drained

8 dried apricots, quartered

Juice of 1 lemon

RECIPE CONTINUES

1   Make the quinoa and vegetables: Preheat the oven to 400°F (205°C).

2   In a small bowl, whisk together the cumin, coriander, ginger, cayenne, and black pepper.

3   In a large bowl, toss together the cauliflower, eggplant, and sweet potato with the oil and half of the spice mix (reserve the other half for the sauce). Arrange the vegetables in an even layer over 2 baking sheets. Roast for 20 minutes, or until the vegetables are tender.

4   Meanwhile, rinse the quinoa under cold running water for 1 minute. Add it to a medium pot with 2 cups (480 ml) of water and bring to a boil. Reduce to a simmer, cover, and cook for 15 to 20 minutes, or until all the water has been absorbed. Turn off the heat and let the quinoa sit for 5 minutes before fluffing with a fork. Set aside.

5   Make the sauce: In a large pot, heat the oil over medium-high heat. When the oil shimmers, add the onion, carrot, and garlic. Season with the salt and reduce the heat to medium-low. Cook until the onion is translucent, about 5 minutes. Stir in the tomatoes, parsley, cilantro, and turmeric along with the reserved spice blend and 1 cup (240 ml) of water. Simmer for 15 to 20 minutes, or until the sauce has thickened. Fold in the kale, chickpeas, and apricots along with the roasted vegetables. Cook for another 5 minutes. Season the sauce with lemon juice and/or more salt, if desired.

6   To serve, place the quinoa in a large serving bowl and top with the vegetable mixture. Garnish with cilantro.

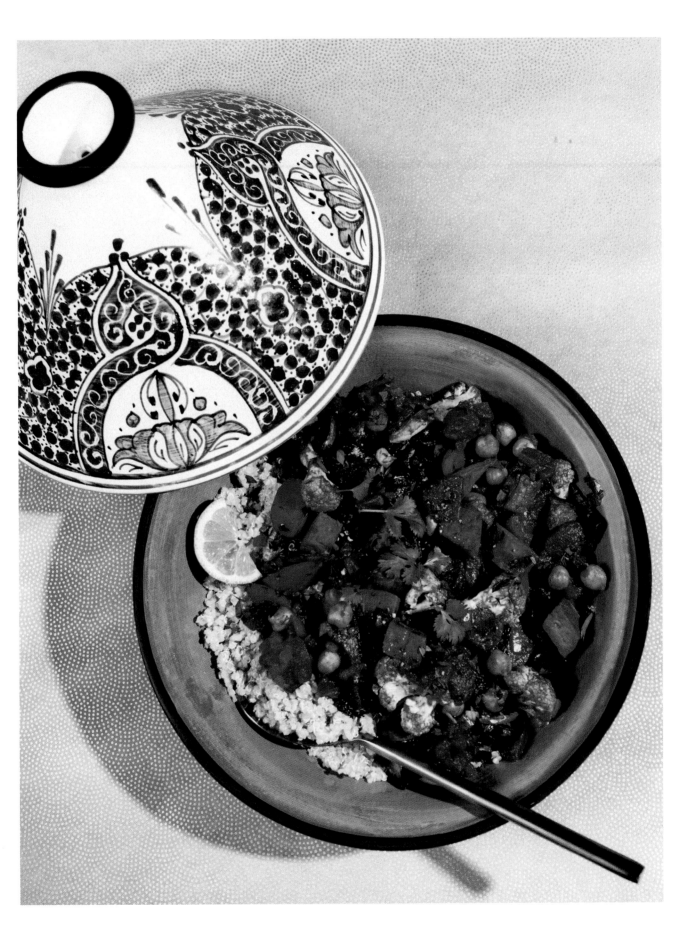

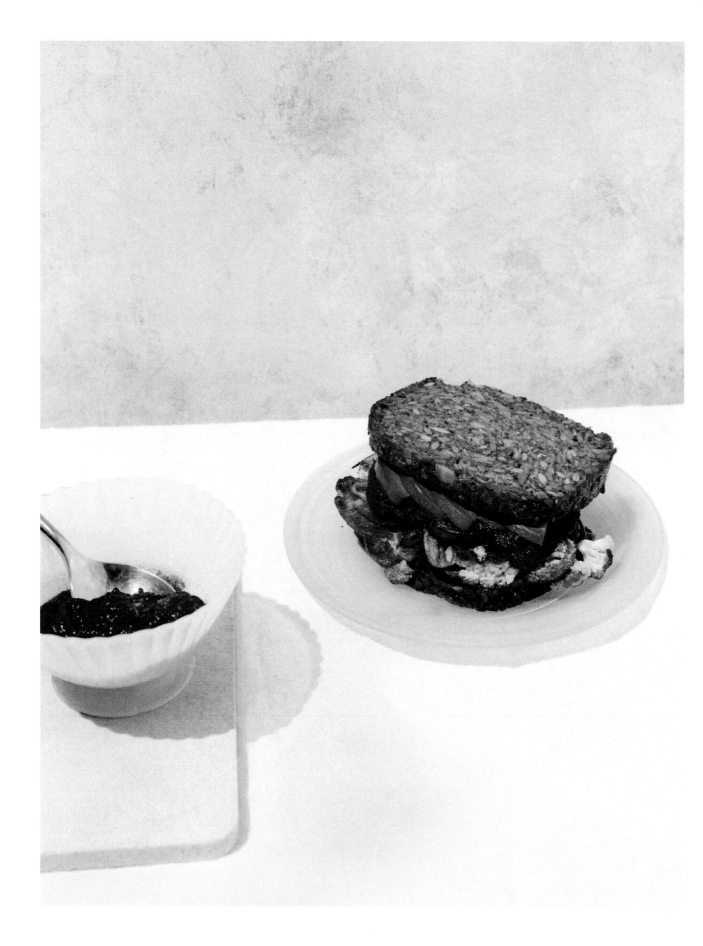

ROASTED CAULIFLOWER STEAK SANDWICHES

FOR THE SMOKY CARROT STEAK SAUCE

½ cup (150 g) grated carrot

½ cup (150 g) grated beet

2 cloves garlic, roughly chopped

1 tablespoon wildflower honey

1 teaspoon smoked paprika

1 teaspoon Himalayan salt

½ teaspoon brown rice vinegar

Freshly ground black pepper

FOR THE STEAK SANDWICH

1 small red onion, cut into 8 wedges

2 tablespoons extra-virgin olive oil

¾ teaspoon Himalayan salt

1 large head cauliflower, cut into 4 slices 1½ inch (4 cm) thick

4 or 8 slices Sakara Seed Bread (page 187), or 4 of your favorite buns

1 avocado, pitted and sliced

1 tomato, sliced

This mega-sandwich proves that plants don't have to be dainty. A slab of thick-sliced cauliflower that's roasted until tender and caramelized gets slathered with a smoky carrot steak sauce and loaded up with crispy onion petals for a nod to a steakhouse favorite. Serve with Daily Greens (page 33) and don't forget a bib. You're welcome!

1   Make the steak sauce: In a small pot, bring 4 cups (960 ml) of water to a boil. Reduce to a simmer and add the carrot and beet. Cook for 10 minutes, or until the vegetables are tender. While they're still hot, thoroughly drain the carrots and beets. Add them to a blender along with the garlic, honey, paprika, salt, vinegar, and ¼ cup (60 ml) of water. Season with a few cracks of pepper and blend until smooth, adding 1 or 2 tablespoons more water if the sauce is too thick. Set aside to cool.

2   Make the cauliflower steaks: Preheat the oven to 400°F (205°C).

3   In a medium bowl, toss the onion petals with 1 tablespoon of the oil and ¼ teaspoon of the salt. Arrange the onion on a baking sheet and roast until caramelized and tender, tossing halfway through, 18 to 20 minutes.

4   On a baking sheet, drizzle the cauliflower slices with the remaining 1 tablespoon of the oil and the remaining ½ teaspoon of salt, using your hands to rub the mixture over both sides of each slice. Roast until the cauliflower is tender and beginning to brown, flipping halfway through, 20 to 25 minutes.

5   Assemble the sandwiches: Top 4 slices of the bread with a cauliflower steak, a drizzle of steak sauce, a tuft of onion petals, a slice of avocado, and a slice of tomato. Enjoy open-faced or top with another slice of bread.

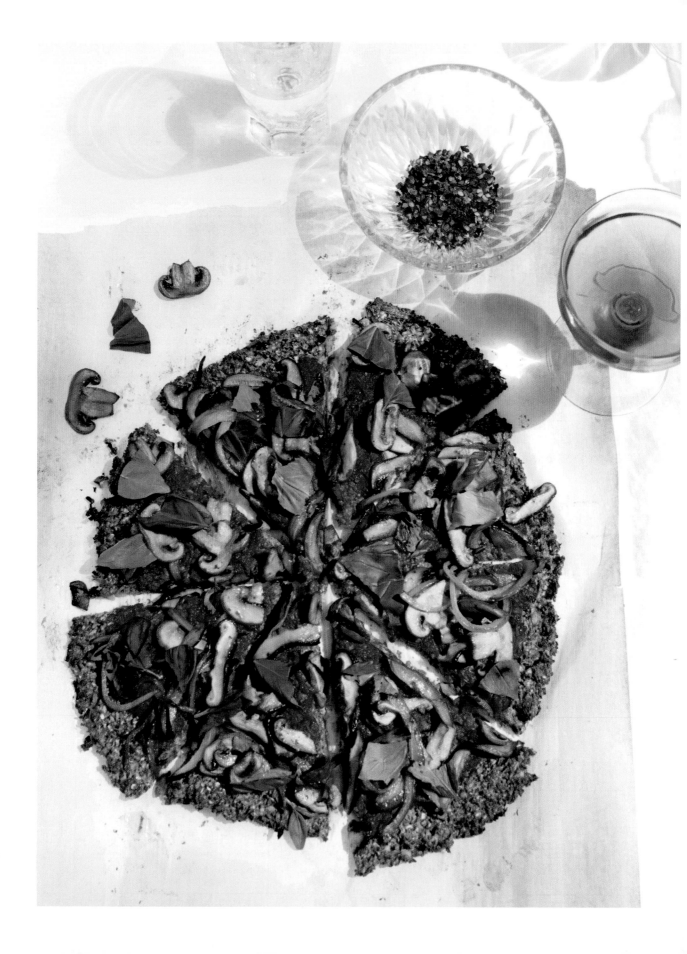

CLASSIC CAULI SLICE

SERVES 4

FOR THE CRUST

½ cup (60 g) ground chia seeds

4 cups (430 g) cauliflower
   florets

½ cup (56 g) quinoa flour or
   (79 g) brown rice flour

1 teaspoon garlic powder

1 teaspoon nutritional yeast

1 teaspoon Himalayan salt

FOR THE TOPPINGS

1 tablespoon extra-virgin
   olive oil

2 cups (150 g) sliced
   mushrooms, such as button,
   shiitake, or oyster

1 cup (100 g) thinly sliced red
   onion

½ cup (120 ml) store-bought
   tomato sauce (use your
   favorite jarred organic
   sauce)

Minced garlic (optional)

Crushed red pepper flakes
   (optional)

½ cup (10 g) fresh basil leaves,
   torn

Cauliflower-crust pizzas bake up just like those with traditional crusts do, all caramelized and crispy, plus you get to indulge in another dose of vegetable healing (without pickier eaters knowing that's what's happening). You can customize this pie any way you like; we love topping ours with plenty of mushrooms and onions—feel free to add some minced garlic and crushed red pepper flakes too, if you're feeling spicy!

1   Make the crust: In a small bowl, whisk the chia seeds with 1½ cups (360 ml) of water. Place the mixture in the refrigerator to set while you work on the cauliflower.

2   Preheat the oven to 450°F (230°C). Place the cauliflower in a food processor and pulse until it reaches a rice-like consistency. Bundle the riced cauliflower in a cheesecloth or dish towel and, standing over the sink or a large bowl, squeeze out any excess liquid. Transfer the drained cauliflower to a large bowl and add the chia mixture, flour, garlic powder, yeast, and salt. Mix the dough thoroughly with your hands or a spoon.

3   Spread the dough about ½ inch (12 mm) thick on a baking sheet in a square or round shape. Bake for 20 minutes, or until the crust is golden brown. Allow the crust to cool for 5 minutes before adding the toppings.

4   Make the toppings: In a large pan, heat the oil over medium heat. Add the mushrooms and onion and sauté until tender, about 3 minutes.

5   Assemble the pizza: Top the crust with the tomato sauce, as well as the minced garlic or crushed red pepper flakes, if using. Add the sautéed vegetables. Place the pizza back in the oven and bake for 8 minutes, or until the crust is golden brown around the edges. Allow the pizza to cool slightly before sprinkling with the basil, slicing, and serving.

SOUTHWESTERN POLENTA CASSEROLE

SERVES 6 TO 8

1 cup (130 g) polenta or corn grits

½ teaspoon Himalayan salt, plus more to taste

Freshly ground black pepper

2 tablespoons extra-virgin olive oil

1 medium yellow onion, chopped

3 cloves garlic, minced

2 cups (350 g) corn kernels, fresh or frozen

2 medium zucchini, diced

1 yellow bell pepper, seeded and diced

1 tablespoon chili powder

1 (14-ounce/400 g) can stewed tomatoes

3 scallions (white and green parts), chopped, for garnish

¼ cup (10 g) chopped cilantro, for garnish

This isn't some sad, throwback dish; when we say *casserole*, we really mean that we've layered up tons of flavors and textures—like corn, another quintessentially summer veg, plus bell pepper, tomatoes, and chili powder to tie it back to our Southwestern roots. Then we top it off with polenta, which lends a sweet creaminess to the dish. It's just the kind of fortification you need after a long day, whether you were hiking the red rocks or scaling the depths of your inbox.

You can buy a roll of ready-made polenta and simply slice and bake, but we recommend taking the extra time (it's not much!) and making it from scratch to avoid any unnecessary additives.

1   Cook the polenta according to the package instructions. Season with the salt and a few cracks of black pepper. Cover and set aside.

2   In a large skillet, heat the oil over medium-high heat. Add the onion and garlic and sauté until the onion begins to get tender and translucent, 3 to 4 minutes. Add the corn, zucchini, bell pepper, and chili powder. Season with a couple of generous pinches of salt and a few cracks of pepper. Cook, stirring occasionally, until the vegetables are tender, 10 to 12 minutes. Stir in the stewed tomatoes and cook just long enough to heat through, 2 to 3 minutes. Taste and add salt, if needed.

3   Preheat the oven to 500°F (260°C).

4   Transfer the mixture to a 9 by 13-inch (23 by 33 cm) baking dish. Dollop the polenta evenly over the top. Bake for 8 to 10 minutes, or until the polenta is heated through and the filling is bubbling. Garnish with the chopped scallions and the cilantro. Serve warm.

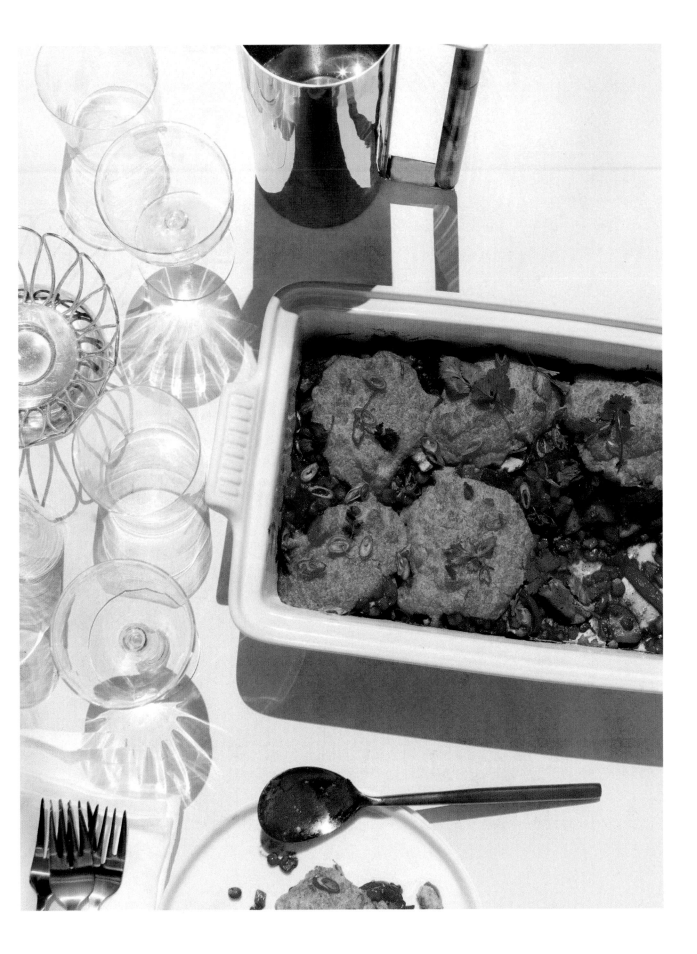

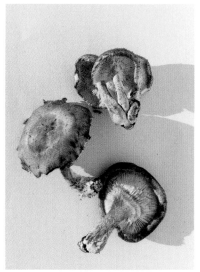
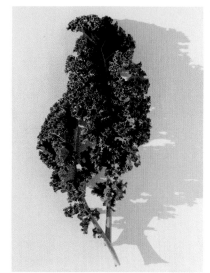
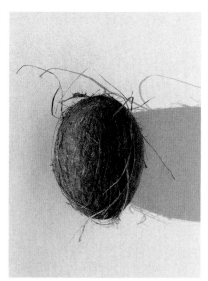
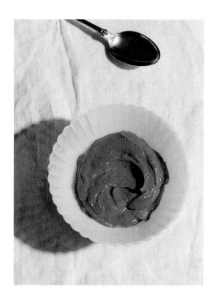

DRESSINGS

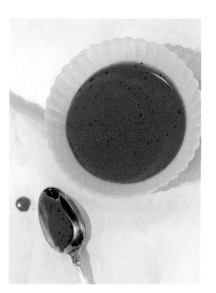
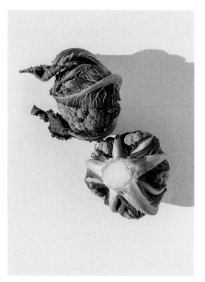
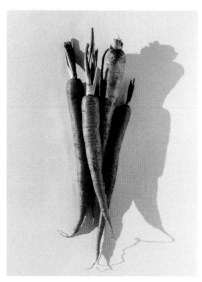
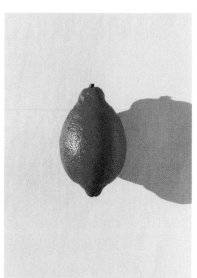

MAPLE + DIJON DRESSING

MAKES ABOUT 1 CUP (240 ML)

¼ cup (60 ml) tahini

¼ cup (60 ml) rice vinegar

¼ cup (60 ml) maple syrup

1 small shallot, minced

1 teaspoon Dijon mustard

½ teaspoon Himalayan salt, or more to taste

2 tablespoons hemp seeds

A drizzle of mineral-rich maple syrup plus spicy Dijon, combined with a sprinkling of protein-packed hemp seeds, make this sweet-savory dressing even more special.

In a blender, combine all the ingredients except the hemp seeds with 2 tablespoons of water. Blend until smooth and stir in the hemp seeds. Store in the fridge for up to 5 days.

TAMARI + LIME VINAIGRETTE

MAKES ABOUT ¾ CUP (180 ML)

¼ cup (60 ml) sesame oil

3 tablespoons tamari soy sauce

Juice of 2 limes

2 teaspoons wildflower honey

1 clove garlic, minced

This bright, bold Asian-inspired vinaigrette is such a client favorite that we had to include it here. It can get even the most veggie-averse folks to fall in love with a salad (or whatever you decide to drizzle it over).

In a jar or medium bowl, combine the ingredients and shake or whisk until smooth. Store in the fridge for up to 5 days.

201

JALAPEÑO + TAHINI DRESSING

½ cup (120 ml) tahini

¼ cup (60 ml) fresh lime juice

½ medium jalapeño, seeded and minced

2 cloves garlic, roughly chopped

1 tablespoon packed fresh cilantro leaves

1 tablespoon chopped fresh ginger

½ teaspoon Himalayan salt

The traditional sesame dressing gets some fresh, green heat.

In a blender, combine all the ingredients with ½ cup (120 ml) of water and blend until smooth. Store in the fridge for up to 5 days.

GREEN GODDESS DRESSING

1 small shallot, roughly chopped

2 cloves garlic, roughly chopped

2 tablespoons brown rice vinegar

1 tablespoon fresh lemon juice

1 tablespoon fresh lime juice

½ bunch fresh cilantro, stems trimmed and roughly chopped

¼ cup (5 g) basil leaves

2 tablespoons mint leaves

1 avocado, pitted and cut into chunks

1 teaspoon Himalayan salt

2 tablespoons extra-virgin olive oil

A fresher, more herbaceous take on the steakhouse classic.

In a blender, combine the shallot, garlic, vinegar, lemon juice, lime juice, cilantro, basil, mint, and avocado and pulse until just combined. Sprinkle in the salt, oil, and ¼ cup (60 ml) of water and blend until smooth. If you want to loosen up the consistency, add additional water.

POPPY SEED DRESSING

MAKES ABOUT 1 CUP (240 ML)

¼ cup (60 ml) plus 1 tablespoon apple cider vinegar

2 tablespoons plus 2 teaspoons wildflower honey

2 tablespoons plus 2 teaspoons Dijon mustard

2 teaspoons poppy seeds

¼ teaspoon Himalayan salt, or more to taste

½ cup (120 ml) sunflower oil

¼ cup (60 ml) plus 1 tablespoon extra-virgin olive oil

The salad bar standby taken to a lighter, brighter place.

In a blender, combine the vinegar, honey, Dijon, poppy seeds, and salt and blend to combine. With the blender running on low speed, slowly stream in the sunflower oil and olive oil until the dressing is creamy and emulsified. Loosen the dressing with 1 or 2 tablespoons of water until you've reached your desired consistency, and season to taste with salt, if desired. Store in the fridge for up to 5 days.

DAYDREAMER DRESSING

SERVES 1

1 tablespoon plus 2 teaspoons tahini

2½ teaspoons brown rice vinegar

2 teaspoons tamari soy sauce

2¼ teaspoons white miso

½ teaspoon sriracha

People have been trying to get their hands on this recipe for years. It is the essential Sakara dressing, and while it may be oil-free, it's nothing short of rich and flavorful thanks to miso and a dash of sriracha. Make a single serving or scale up for a week's worth.

In a jar, combine all the ingredients with 2 tablespoons of water. Shake well until completely combined.

DRESSINGS

203

GINGER + TURMERIC DRESSING

MAKES ABOUT ¾ CUP (180 ML)

3 tablespoons tahini

Juice of 1½ limes

1 tablespoon grated fresh ginger

1 tablespoon roughly chopped fresh cilantro leaves

2 teaspoons wildflower honey

½ teaspoon Himalayan salt, or more to taste

¼ teaspoon ground turmeric

Two anti-inflammatory powerhouses join forces for one gorgeously golden dressing.

In a blender, combine all the ingredients with ¼ cup (60 ml) plus 2 tablespoons of water. Blend until smooth. Taste and add more salt, if desired. Store in the fridge for up to 5 days.

GREEN CITRUS DRESSING

MAKES ABOUT 1½ CUPS (360 ML)

1 cup (25 g) fresh mint leaves

1 cup (20 g) fresh basil leaves

½ cup (25 g) fresh cilantro leaves and stems

1 medium avocado, pitted and peeled

1 small shallot, roughly chopped

2½ tablespoons fresh lemon juice

2 tablespoons extra-virgin olive oil

1 tablespoon fresh orange juice

1 tablespoon fresh lime juice

2 teaspoons Champagne vinegar

1 clove garlic, roughly chopped

¼ teaspoon Himalayan salt, or more to taste

With its fresh mint and basil plus orange juice and Champagne vinegar, this dressing is like a garden party in a jar.

In a blender, combine all the ingredients with ¼ cup (60 ml) of water and blend until smooth. Add additional water, 1 tablespoon at a time, to thin the consistency, if desired. Season to taste with salt. Store in the fridge for up to 3 days.

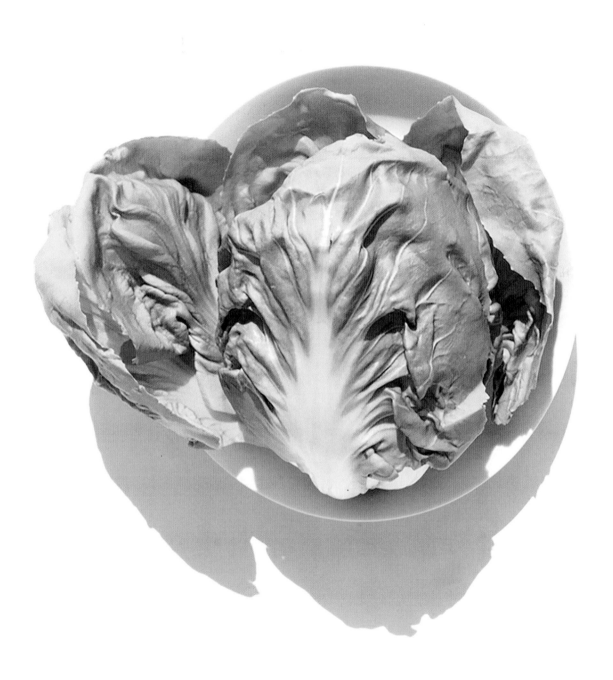

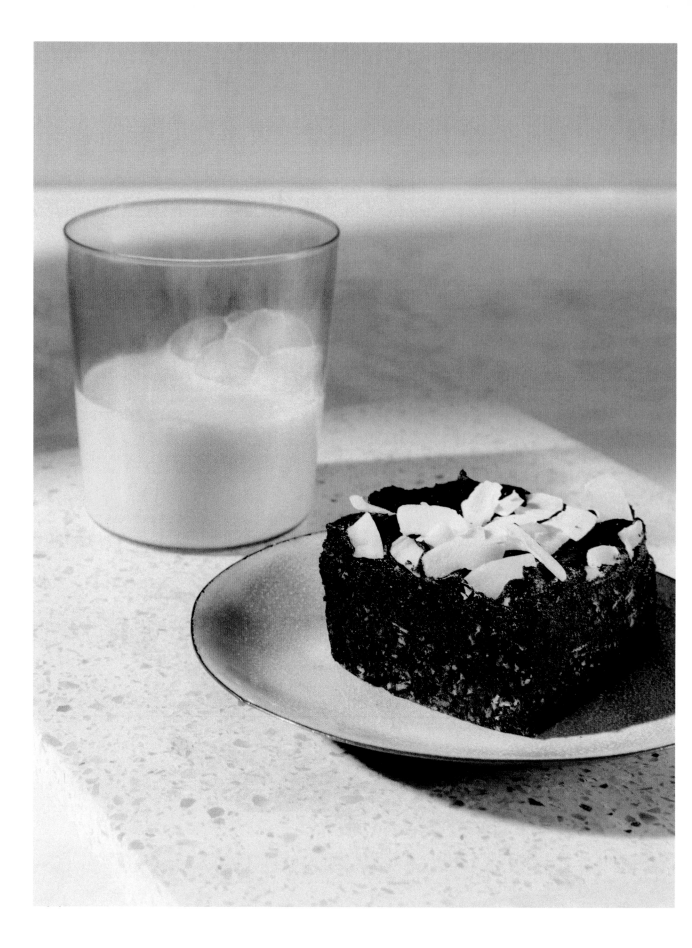

Desserts

When it comes to balanced, vibrant health, sweetness is just as important to embrace as any other flavor. But when creating something sweet, we balance it with the goodness of whole foods, fiber, protein, and superfoods. This way it can be another amazing form of getting nutrients into the body—as well as love.

CACAO POWER BROWNIES, *following page*

CACAO POWER BROWNIES

MAKES 24 BROWNIES

FOR THE BROWNIES

2 cups (350 g) pitted dates

1¼ cups (140 g) packed
    almond flour

¾ cup (75 g) raw cacao powder

3 tablespoons shelled hemp
    seeds

1 teaspoon Himalayan salt

2 cups (200 g) rolled oats

1 cup (100 g) raw walnuts

3¼ cups (275 g) unsweetened
    shredded coconut

½ cup (120 ml) plus
    1 tablespoon maple syrup

½ cup (120 ml) unsweetened
    almond milk

2 teaspoons pure vanilla extract

FOR THE GANACHE AND TOPPING

¾ cup (180 ml) maple syrup

1 cup (100 g) raw cacao powder

2 tablespoons maca powder

2 cups (170 g) shredded
    coconut flakes

These dense, fudgy brownies with a maple-cacao ganache are decadent enough to serve as dessert, but their high plant protein content, thanks to oats, hemp seeds, and almonds, makes them a perfectly acceptable—and encouraged—breakfast. Pro tip: Adding a dose of adaptogens (powdered superherbs) to the ganache is a great way to get in some extra healing. We love maca for this because it's a sweet, malty-flavored root that actively helps your body adapt to stressors while giving you a natural boost of energy and an even-keeled lifting of the spirits.

1   Make the brownies: In a medium bowl, soak the dates for 20 minutes in enough boiling water to cover. Line a 9 by 13-inch (23 by 33 cm) pan with parchment paper and set aside.

2   In a large bowl, mix together the flour, cacao powder, hemp seeds, and salt. Set aside.

3   In a food processor, pulse together the oats, walnuts, and shredded coconut until they are the texture of coarse meal. Add this mixture to the flour mixture and set aside.

4   Drain the dates and add them to a blender along with the maple syrup, milk, and vanilla. Blend until completely combined, then add the mixture to the dry ingredients. Stir until the batter is evenly combined.

5   Press the batter evenly in the prepared pan, gently pressing it down with your spoon or spatula.

6   Make the ganache: In a blender, combine the maple syrup, cacao, and maca and blend until smooth. Pour the glaze over the brownies. Sprinkle the coconut flakes evenly over the glaze. Refrigerate the brownies overnight to set. Slice into roughly 2 by 2-inch (5 by 5 cm) squares and serve. Store leftovers in the fridge for up to 5 days.

CACAO

Cacao

ENHANCES

YOUR ABILITY TO

find your bliss

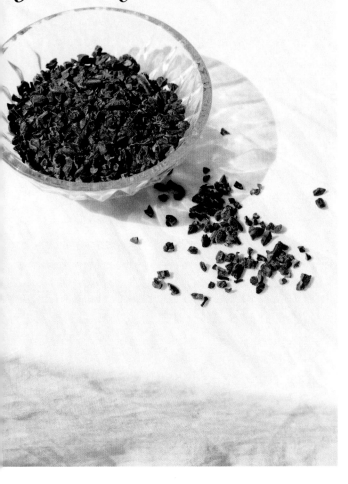

THE MAYANS WERE ON TO SOMETHING IN BELIEVING THAT CACAO HAD LEGENDARY POWERS.

In its raw, unprocessed state, cacao is a potent superfood, filled with beautiful, health-enhancing, vibrant properties that will make you glow from the inside out. It boasts the highest number of antioxidants of any whole food in the world, protecting against toxins in your body and helping prevent disease, while its flavonoids promote cardiovascular health by improving circulation and blood pressure. Cacao is also a significant source of magnesium, a vital nutrient that the majority of us Americans are deficient in. Magnesium works to balance the chemistry of your brain by acting as a muscle relaxant, reducing the harmful effects of stress and encouraging a restful night's sleep. It also helps keep bones healthy and strong by assisting in the absorption of calcium. And cacao is packed with a variety of neurotransmitters that work as natural antidepressants, enhancing your ability to focus and increasing pleasure and bliss.

DESSERTS

209

TURMERIC + MEYER LEMON SQUARES

FOR THE CRUST

1¾ cups (165 g) almond meal

½ cup (70 g) tapioca flour

¼ cup (60 ml) coconut oil, melted

¼ cup (60 ml) maple syrup

FOR THE FILLING

⅓ cup (75 ml) freshly squeezed Meyer lemon juice (about 1½ lemons)

2 tablespoons cornstarch

1 cup (240 ml) full-fat coconut milk

⅓ cup (75 ml) maple syrup

2 tablespoons coconut oil

½ teaspoon ground turmeric

½ teaspoon pure vanilla extract

Zest of ½ Meyer lemon or regular lemon

½ Meyer lemon, thinly sliced

Even in the grayest, coldest winter, there lays the promise of sunshine. Just when we need its bright alchemy, citrus starts popping up at the market to announce that in just a few months we'll be back standing in the sun. One of our favorites is the Meyer lemon, a hybrid fruit native to China. It's essentially a cross between a lemon and a mandarin orange, giving it a floral flavor with a pleasant pucker (and a lemon's signature dose of cold-combatting vitamin C). We've also added a hit of anti-inflammatory golden child turmeric to make this one part dessert, one part winter tool-kit essential.

If you can't find Meyer lemons near you, substitute one-half tangerine or grapefruit and one-half lemon.

1   Make the crust: Preheat the oven to 350°F (175°C). Line an 8-inch-square (20 cm) pan with parchment paper and set aside.

2   In a large bowl, whisk together the almond meal and tapioca flour until combined. Stir in the oil and maple syrup and mix until combined. Press the mixture into the bottom of the pan and bake until the crust is lightly browned around the edges, 15 to 20 minutes.

3   Make the filling: In a medium pot, whisk together the lemon juice and cornstarch until no lumps remain. Whisk in all the remaining ingredients except the lemon slices.

4   Bring the mixture to a simmer over medium heat, stirring frequently, until the filling thickens, about 8 minutes. Remove from the heat and let cool for 10 minutes.

5   Pour the filling over the crust and refrigerate for 3 hours, or until completely set. Lift the bars out of the pan and cut into 16 squares. Top each with a slice of lemon and serve.

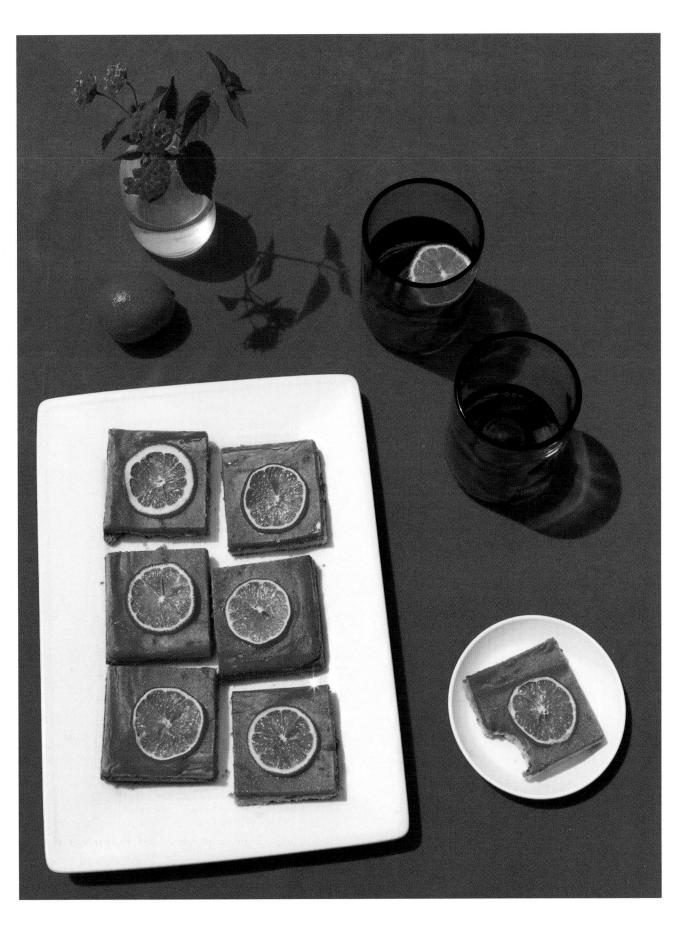

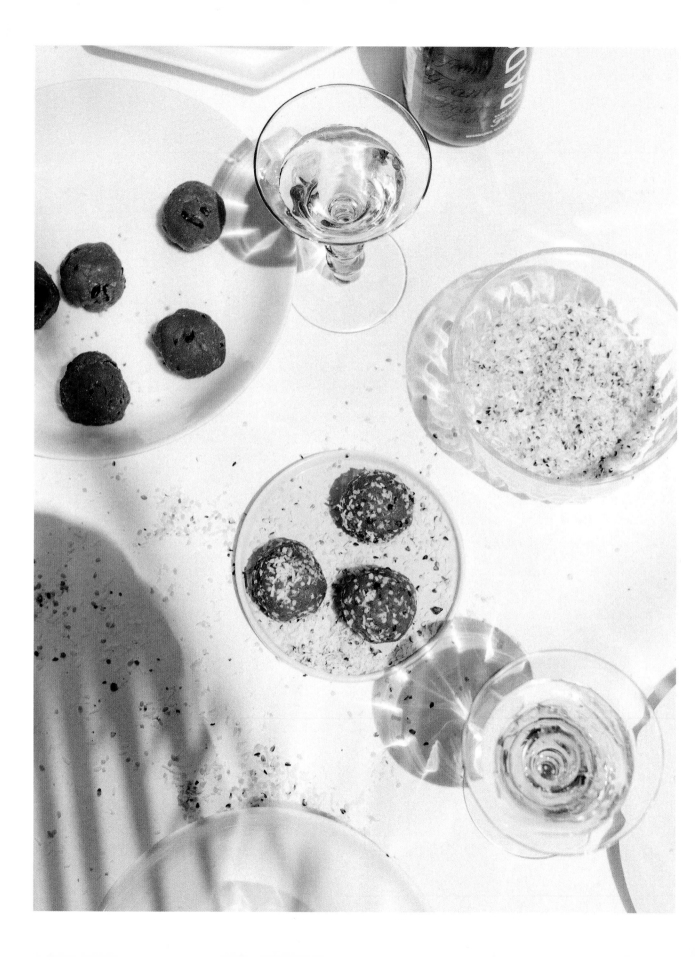

SUPERFOOD COOKIE DOUGH BITES

½ cup (120 ml) almond butter

¼ cup (60 ml) maple syrup

½ teaspoon pure vanilla extract

¼ cup (30 g) coconut flour

3 tablespoons flaxseed meal

¼ teaspoon Himalayan salt

¼ cup (30 g) cacao nibs

2 tablespoons hemp seeds

2 tablespoons unsweetened
	shredded coconut

We've rolled up three of our favorite superfoods—cacao nibs, flaxseed, and hemp seeds—into one sweet, doughy little nibble. They're a perfectly suitable indulgence any time of day, whether it's après dinner or avant lunch.

1   In a large bowl, stir together the almond butter, maple syrup, and vanilla until creamy. In a medium bowl, combine the flour, flaxseed meal, and salt.

2   Add the dry ingredients to the wet and mix well to combine. Use the back of your spoon to work in the cacao nibs. Use your hands to roll the dough into 1-inch (2.5 cm) balls.

3   In a small bowl or on a plate, mix together the hemp seeds and shredded coconut. Roll each ball in the mixture until fully coated. Refrigerate the bites for at least 30 minutes before serving. Store leftovers in the fridge for up to 1 week, or in the freezer for up to 1 month.

DESSERTS

SEED BUTTER COOKIES

⅓ cup (30 g) oat flour

½ cup (130 g) sunflower seed butter

2 tablespoons wildflower honey

¼ cup (35 g) sunflower seeds

¼ teaspoon baking soda

⅛ teaspoon baking powder

½ teaspoon pure vanilla extract

Pinch of Himalayan salt

These bite-size cookies throw it back to a simpler time when a couple of tiny treats in your lunchbox could brighten your day. They're soft, chewy, and satisfyingly nutty, and are made with school-friendly (tree nut-free) sunflower seed butter.

1   In a large bowl, combine all the ingredients and mix until smooth. Cover the bowl with plastic wrap and refrigerate the dough overnight.

2   Preheat the oven to 350°F (175°C). Line a baking sheet with parchment paper or a silicone baking mat.

3   Portion out the dough into 1-tablespoon-size balls. Arrange the cookies on the prepared baking sheet about 2 inches (5 cm) apart. Gently press on each ball to flatten it slightly, then use a fork to create a crosshatch pattern on top. Bake until the cookies are lightly browned around the edges, about 7 minutes. Let the cookies cool slightly before transferring them to the fridge to cool completely, which will prevent the cookies from getting too crumbly. Store the cookies in an airtight container at room temperature for up to 1 week.

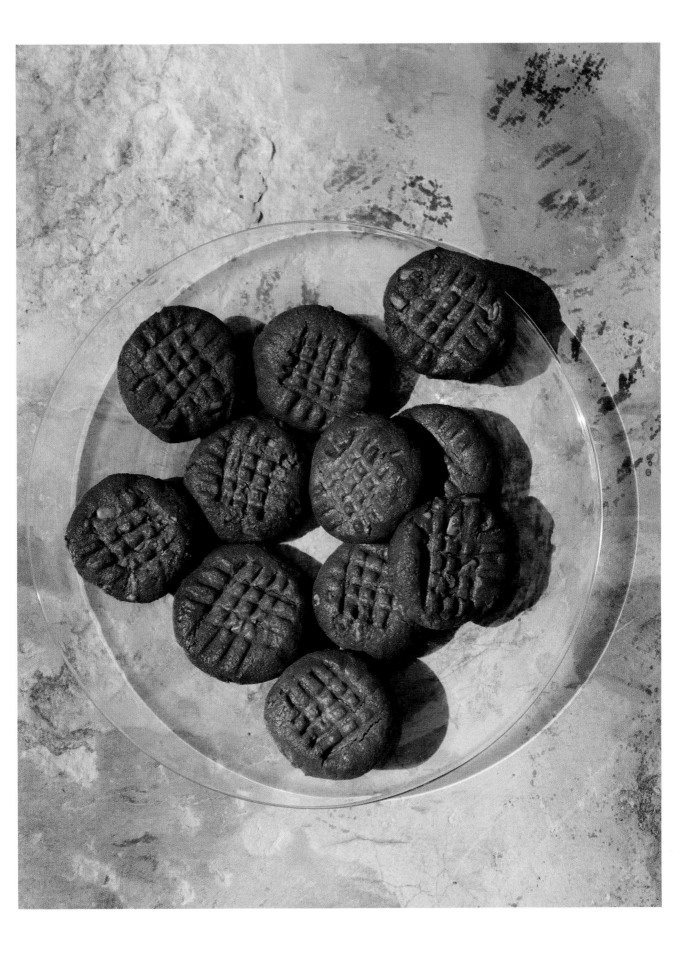

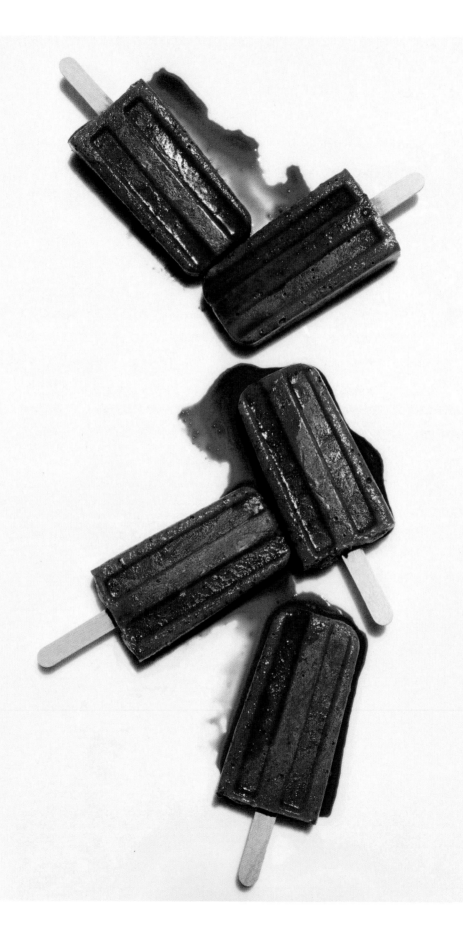

STRAWBERRY + CHIA-SICLES

MAKES ABOUT 12 LARGE
OR 18 SMALL POPS

3 cups (430 g) fresh or frozen strawberries (about 1 pound), stemmed

1 (13½-ounce/400 ml) can full-fat coconut milk

½ medium beet, peeled and diced

3 tablespoons maple syrup

2 tablespoons chia seeds

½ teaspoon pure vanilla extract

10 dropperfuls Sakara Beauty Water Concentrate (optional)

Maybe it's because they're members of the rose family (little-known fact!), or maybe it's because their perfumed flavor reminds us of childhood summers and pink-stained fingers, but we're particularly fond of sweet, succulent strawberries. It doesn't hurt that they're also one of our favorite ways to build beauty from the inside, providing the cells with plumping hydration and antiaging polyphenol protection. We love blending them into this chilled treat, along with healing heavyweights beets and chia seeds. To get the most flavor from your fruit, we recommend using berries at peak freshness and ripeness. And for a rosy finish—and a mineral boost—add some of our Sakara Beauty Water Concentrate (which can be found on our website, Sakara.com).

In a blender, combine all the ingredients and blend on high until smooth. Pour the mixture into ice pop molds. Insert sticks and freeze for 2 to 3 hours, or until completely frozen. Store in the freezer for up to 1 month.

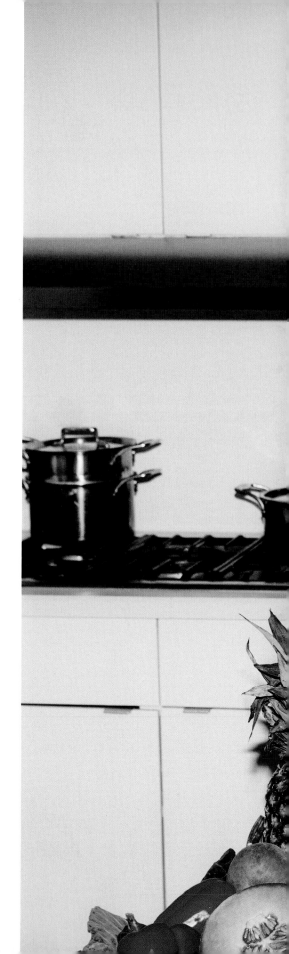

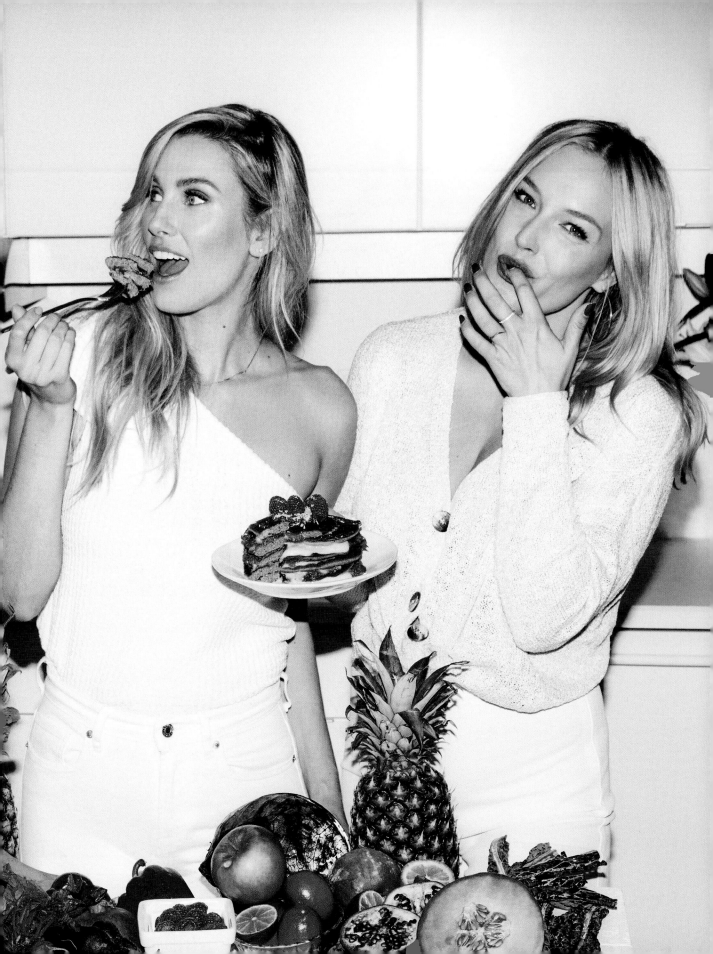

STRAWBERRY + COCONUT CREAM DOUGHNUTS

MAKES 10 DOUGHNUTS

FOR THE STRAWBERRY GLAZE

6 large strawberries (the riper the better)

½ cup (120 ml) coconut cream

¼ cup (60 ml) coconut oil, melted

1 teaspoon maple syrup

FOR THE DOUGHNUTS

1⅔ cups (260 g) gluten-free all-purpose flour

½ cup (95 g) coconut palm sugar

¼ cup (35 g) crushed dried strawberries

1 tablespoon ground flaxseed

1 teaspoon baking powder

1 cup (240 ml) unsweetened nut milk (we prefer almond)

¼ cup (60 ml) coconut oil

1 teaspoon pure vanilla extract

Dehydrated strawberries, for garnish

Practicing self-love means connecting with the sweetness of self-compassion—embracing freedom, expansion, and balance. Let these doughnuts remind you that true love comes in many forms and is best enjoyed with an open heart.

1   Make the strawberry glaze: In a blender, combine all the ingredients and blend until smooth. Chill the glaze in the fridge for at least 45 minutes or overnight.

2   Make the doughnuts: Preheat the oven to 325°F (165°C). Lightly grease 12 doughnut molds and set aside.

3   In a large bowl, combine the flour, sugar, dried strawberries, flaxseed, and baking powder. Set aside.

4   In a small saucepan, gently warm the milk and oil over medium-low heat until the oil is melted and the milk is warm to the touch. Remove from the heat and stir in the vanilla.

5   Fold the milk mixture into the dry ingredients and stir until smooth. Pour the batter into the prepared doughnut molds. Bake until golden and firm to the touch, 18 minutes.

6   Allow the doughnuts to cool completely in the molds. Flip them over and gently tap the bottom of the molds with a spoon to ease the doughnuts from the pan. Use a spoon to drizzle the doughnuts with the strawberry glaze, sprinkle with the dehydrated strawberries, and serve.

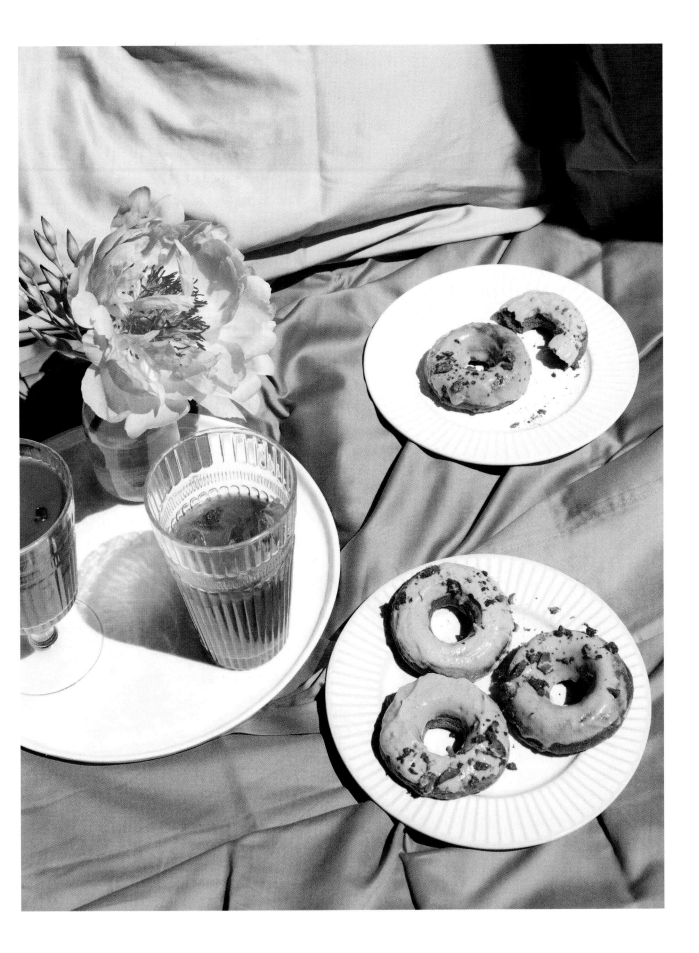

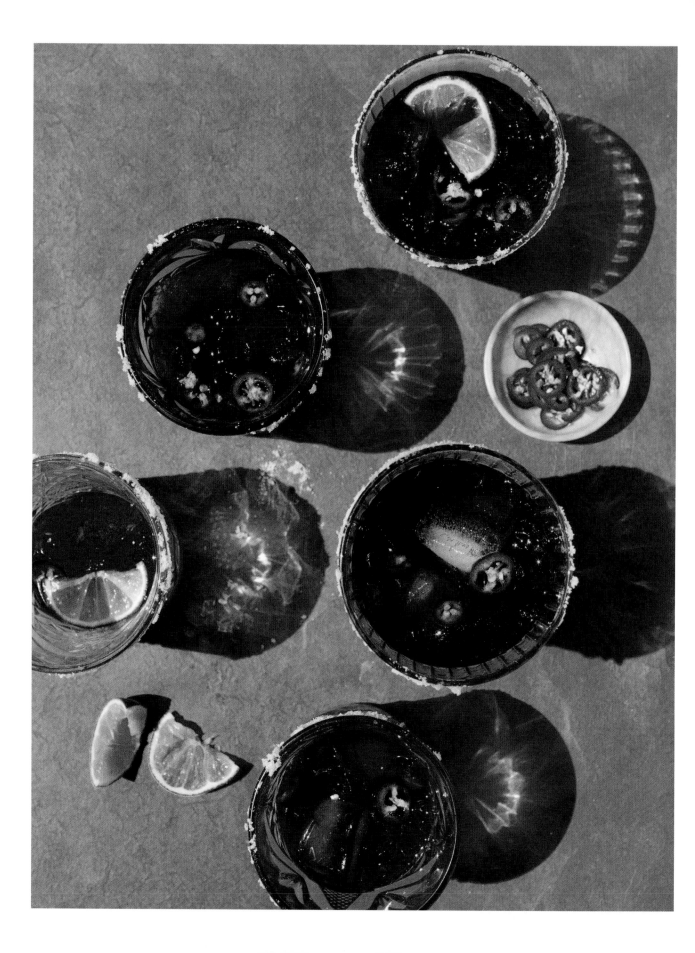

Cocktails We believe life is about balance. That it should be filled with joyous times, including the occasional spirited indulgence. These recipes are our go-to elixirs for when we want to take a walk on the wild side—without dulling our glow.

THE DESERT ROSE, *following page*

THE DESERT ROSE

⅓ jalapeño, seeded and thinly sliced, plus more for garnish

1½ ounces (45 ml/1 shot) mezcal

2 limes, 1 thinly sliced

2 to 3 tablespoons cold-pressed juice (we like a beet-fruit blend for color)

5 dropperfuls of Sakara Beauty Water Concentrate

Splash of club soda or seltzer

Liquid sweetener of choice (we like stevia)

Nature's wisdom has shown us that a flower can bloom even in the desert, which to us means that we can all flourish under the harshest conditions—like stress or work-life imbalance. Taking a moment to celebrate even the smallest victories (such as making it through the week in one piece!) reenergizes the spirit. And doing so with a spicy, smoky beverage made with restorative foods and compounds? Even better.

This drink features our Beauty Water Concentrate, which delivers seventy-two trace minerals, including silica (one of the minerals that our bodies need most and that supports healthy, glowing hair and skin), in addition to rose water. If you don't have our Beauty Water Concentrate (from our website, Sakara.com), you can use organic rose water to give a similar essence of rose to the drink.

In a cocktail shaker or tall glass, muddle the jalapeño. Fill the shaker or glass with ice, then add the mezcal, 1 tablespoon of lime juice, the pressed juice, and Beauty Water Concentrate. Shake well and strain into a glass over fresh ice. Top with a splash of club soda and adjust the sweetness to your liking. Garnish with a couple of slices of lime and jalapeño.

ROSE WATER

DRINK *rose water* AND FALL IN *love*

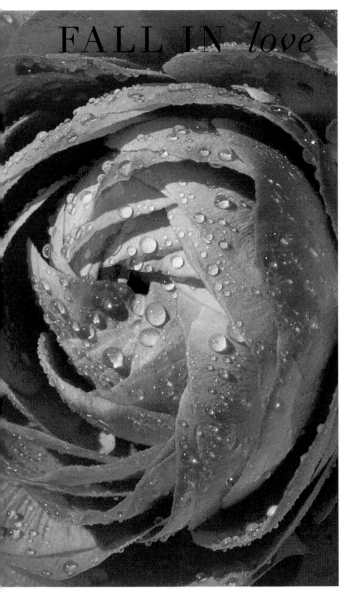

ROSE WATER IS ONE OF THE ORIGINAL BEAUTY FOODS, USED BY THE ROMANS AND THE MOST NOTORIOUS GODDESS HERSELF, CLEOPATRA.

With its sultry floral fragrance, rose water is also a natural healer that can lower stress and anxiety; deliver vitamins A, B_3, C, D, and E; repair aging skin; and lift your mood. And it contains a chemical called phenylethylamine, which is what the brain produces when you're in love . . . and after a little sexy time. We add a splash to water or tea, smoothies, and even desserts.

When buying rose water, look for "distilled" and "organic" on the label in order to avoid buying a synthetic product or one that contains preservatives.

COCKTAILS

225

SEDONA SUNSET MARGARITA

¼ cup (60 ml) mezcal

2 tablespoons juiced turmeric root

1 tablespoon freshly squeezed orange juice

1 tablespoon agave nectar

1 lime

Lime wedges

1 teaspoon coarse Himalayan salt

1 teaspoon ground turmeric

Orange zest, for garnish

Sunsets are a magical moment. A marking of time, and an energetic shift in the day. This margarita is an ode to our Sedona roots, where the margarita is the unofficial cocktail and where the sunsets over the red rocks remind us of the possibility of something greater than ourselves. As we know that anything you put into your body can be a vehicle for extra nutrients—cocktails included—we've added a dash of turmeric for its anti-inflammatory and health benefits. We use this cocktail potion as a tonic to enter the evening hours with a peaceful body and mind. And to open ourselves to what the night may have in store. . . ! If you can't juice your own turmeric root, one teaspoon of ground turmeric will work just as well. Simply increase the orange juice to 3 tablespoons.

1   Fill a cocktail shaker with ice and add the mezcal, turmeric, orange juice, agave nectar, and the juice of ½ lime. Shake well.

2   On a small plate, mix together the salt and ground turmeric.

3   Run a lime wedge around the rim of a glass, then dip the rim in the salt and turmeric mixture.

4   Serve the margarita over ice. Garnish with a strip of orange zest, a lime wedge, and visions of gorgeous pink and purple skies.

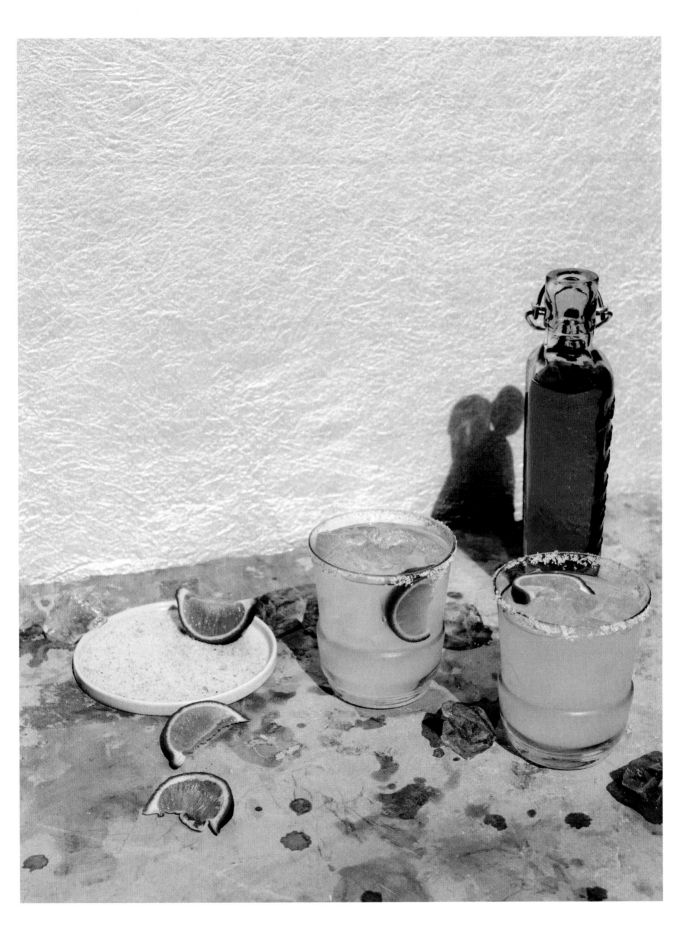

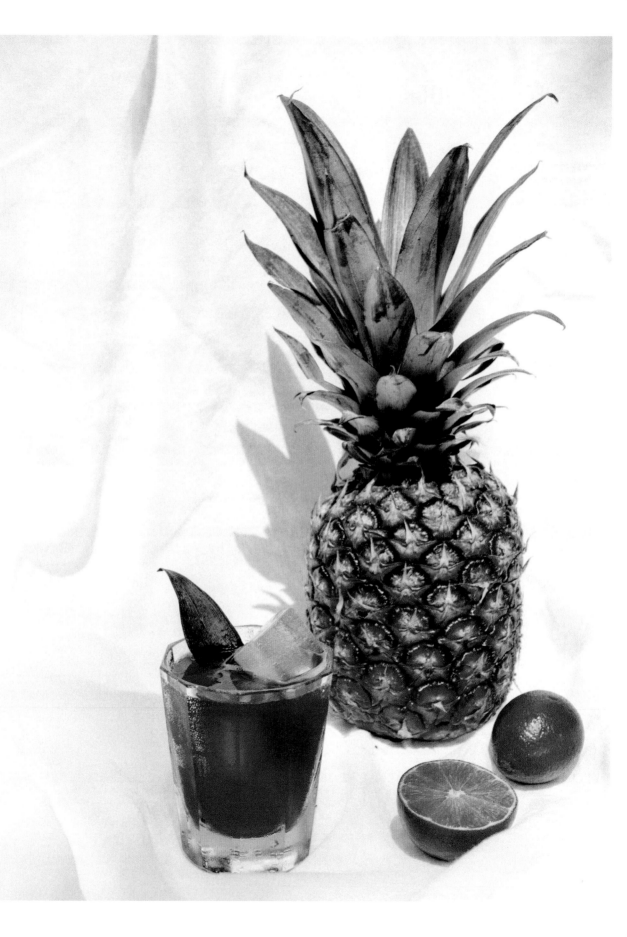

GINGER KOMBUCHA MULE

MAKES 1 COCKTAIL

¾ cup (180 ml) ginger
   kombucha (we love
   Health-Ade)

2 ounces (60 ml) vodka

Juice of 1 lime

Splash of pineapple juice

1 teaspoon molasses

Pineapple leaf, for garnish

For summertime sipping, we took a traditional Moscow Mule and gave it a Sakara glow. We swapped out the ginger beer for ginger kombucha, one of our favorite fermented botanicals. Since about two thousand years ago, in Asia, this magic potion has been dubbed the "immortal health elixir" because of its ability to support body-wide health and prevent illnesses. High-quality kombucha is filled with probiotics and amino acids that help your body digest sugars, and also happens to be a natural hangover cure. A match made in cocktail heaven!

In a tall glass, combine the kombucha, vodka, lime juice, pineapple juice, and molasses and stir. Garnish with the pineapple leaf and enjoy.

VANILLA + MEYER LEMON GIN AND TONIC

FOR THE VANILLA BEAN SYRUP

1 cup (240 ml) wildflower
    honey

1 vanilla bean

FOR THE COCKTAIL

2 tablespoons freshly squeezed
    Meyer lemon juice

2 ounces (60 ml) gin

½ cup (120 ml) tonic water

Edible flowers, for garnish

We gave this classic cocktail an extra-refreshing yet sensual twist by adding a squeeze of perfumed Meyer lemon juice and a vanilla-infused simple syrup to stir the senses and arouse the spirit. Ever since the Aztecs enjoyed their signature vanilla-scented, love-inducing elixir *chocolatl*, this fragrant pod has been notorious for its naughty charms. When the Europeans got their hands on the spice, doctors began prescribing it to stimulate the appetite (they weren't talking about dinner), and women began dabbing it behind their ears to draw an admirer's gaze. As you sip this beverage, invite your senses to play.

If you can't find Meyer lemons, use one-half tangerine or grapefruit juice and one-half lemon juice.

1   Make the vanilla syrup: In a small pot, combine the honey with 1 cup (240 ml) of water. Slice the vanilla bean down the center and scrape out the seeds into the pot, then add the pod. Heat over medium-high heat, stirring occasionally, until the sugar has dissolved completely and the mixture has come to a boil, 10 to 15 minutes. Remove from the heat and pour into a jar. Let the syrup cool completely before using. Store any leftover syrup in the fridge for up to 1 week.

2   Make the cocktail: In a shaker, add a handful of ice and pour over the lemon juice, gin, and 1 to 2 tablespoons of the vanilla syrup, to taste. Shake vigorously and strain into a highball glass. Add the tonic and ice to fill the glass, then garnish with the flowers.

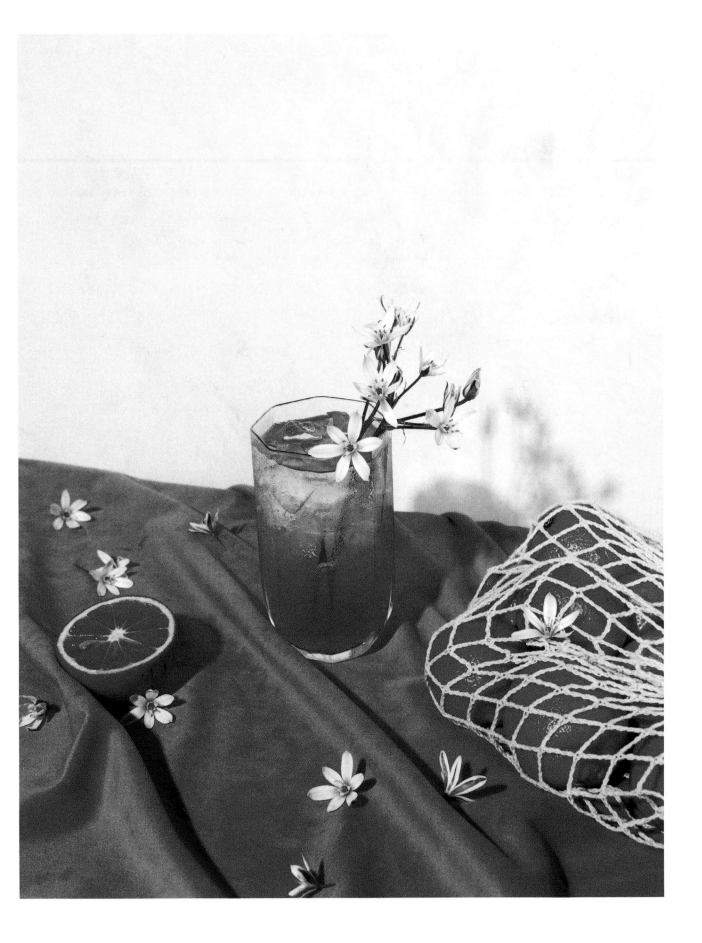

HONEYDEW + LYCHEE SPRITZER

¼ cup (45 g) honeydew melon,
    plus 1 slice for garnish

2 lychees

½ cup (120 ml) of your favorite
    white wine

Sparkling water

Edible flowers, for garnish

We believe that anything you put in your body is an opportunity to deliver healing, so we wanted to create a cocktail that actually provides hydration—not the norm for adult beverages. By adding quenching honeydew melon and vitamin C–rich lychee, we turned basic white wine into a refresher for body and soul.

In a shaker, muddle the melon and lychees until the melon is broken down and smooth. Add the wine and shake. Fill a wineglass three-quarters full with ice for a large glass, or half full for a small glass. Pour the wine mixture over the top. Add a splash of sparkling water and a slice of melon, and garnish with flowers. Enjoy.

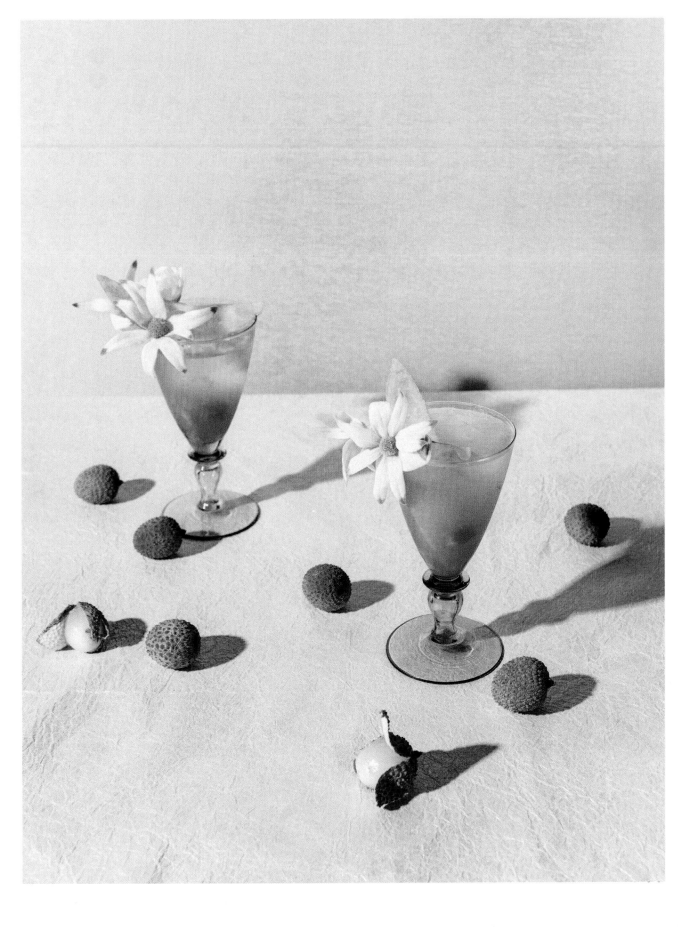

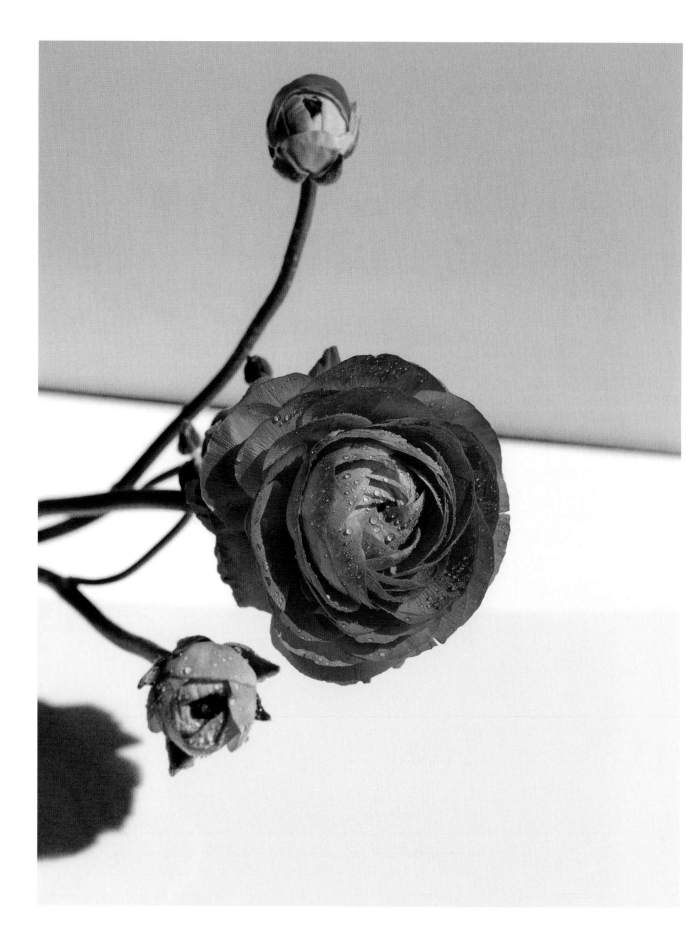

DESSERT AFTER DESSERT: LOVE OIL

As you know by now, we're all about keeping it clean, even when we're playing dirty. This includes our…extracurricular activities. But just because our evenings (and some mornings, and afternoons too) can get a little naughty does *not* mean that our products should be. Nurturing your relationships is a crucial part of a balanced life because these connections help us feel grounded and supported, bring us joy, and in some special cases, pleasure. And getting physically intimate with your partner is just as nourishing as eating your greens! It strengthens the immune system, soothes the nervous system, supports heart health, rejuvenates the spirit, and even eases pain. So whipping up a batch of this massage oil/personal lubricant is just as much an act of self-care as making any other recipe in this book. We especially love this concoction because it's free of any of the harmful ingredients that you'll find in many conventional products. Instead, there's kitchen-staple coconut oil plus sweet almond oil for extra skin nourishment from vitamins A and E. And you can customize it depending on which essential oils really do it for you—peppermint for a tingly, cooling sensation, lavender for calming, bergamot for sexy and floral. Choose your own adventure. Just one FYI: Oil-based lubes can degrade latex, so if using this as personal lubricant it's best to reserve it for a monogamous, fluid-bonded partnership where there's no concern about STIs or pregnancy. Now go forth and find your bliss!

MAKES 1 BATCH

Mix equal parts organic coconut oil and organic sweet almond oil. Add a drop or two of essential oils, if desired. Store in a lidded container at room temperature and use clean hands or a spoon to remove from the jar. If you live somewhere cold during the winter (like New York City), the oils may solidify, but the warmth from your body will cause them to liquify it again.

ACKNOWLEDGMENTS AND THANK-YOUS

Rachel Holtzman, *writer*

Kirby Stirland, *copywriter*

Gabby Lester-Coll, *copywriter*

Lianna Tarantin, *photographer*

Caitlin Mitchell, *portraits*

Pearl Jones, *food stylist*

Anna Niedermeyer, *prop stylist*

Erin Cauley, *stylist and photo assistant*

Melanie Grigonis, *project manager*

Deb Wood, *art director*

Holly Dolce, *editor*

Tyler Harvey, *r+d chef*

A special thank you to Joshua and Cristina Abrams for so generously
opening their beautiful home to us for the setting of this book.
And to Mattias Stanghed for being one of our first clients
and pushing us to go further.